Rays of Grace

A Story of Strength and Spirit

By
Melinda Ferreira

"In Rays of Grace: A Story of Strength & Spirit, Melinda Ferreira writes with great clarity, honesty and passionate good humor about her mother, Marian Ciampa. It is hard not to fall in love with Marian, whose presence and absence fill this book. Ferreira lovingly reveals the gifts and the challenges presented to her and her family through the illness and death of her mother. This is an unflinchingly brave book that talks about the pain of losing a mother at the age of 14, while chronicling the author's own resilience as she anticipates her mother's death and the shattering of her world. In celebrating the life of a complex and imperfect person, Melinda opens our hearts to her mother while maintaining a writer's eye for the lessons of loss carried and transformed. Like all great writing, the specifics of one life lead us to a deeper truth that resonates within all of us. An outstanding read."

—Paul Golding, MBA
President, National Alliance for Grieving Children

"The honesty with which Melinda Ferreira writes is deeply affecting. *Rays of Grace* is a poignant account of the strength and love of the author's family as it endures the heartache of her mother's struggles with alcoholism and breast cancer. Ferreira brings us intimately into her life, and we come to adore her mother through the eyes of a child. We can all take something away from the spiritual honesty of Melinda and her mother Marian."

—Gayun Chan-Smutko, MS
Genetic Counselor
Massachusetts General Hospital, Boston, MA

"This book captivates throughout. Ferreira writes with incredibly intimate detail about the painful issues that often surround disease and addiction. Proving to be a true storyteller, she creates an environment which allows readers to feel as though they are sitting right next to her as she narrates; cheering her on, laughing, crying, feeling her joy and her pain. The love and respect between mother and daughter is beautifully apparent as you go along this journey with Melinda. Regardless of circumstance: whether readers have endured similar situations, or if they have experienced loss or hardship on a different level, *Rays of Grace* manages to relate to a wide range of individuals.

The passion, spirit, and determination displayed by the author's mother, in the face of adversity, have emblazoned Ferreira with an enlightened perspective on life and the meaning within. *Rays of Grace* reminds us of the gifts we so often forget, and awakens its readers to the possibility of finding hope in every circumstance. This book will open readers' minds to the interconnected nature of graces we bestow upon one another, and the impact it has on our paths."

—Teresa Hallquist
Assistant Tour Manager
FUZE-Susan G Komen 2008 National Tour

"*Rays of Grace* captures the innate, primitive, and special bond which exists between a mother and her daughter, both in life and in death. Readers will be inspired and captivated by the mother's passionate yet stoic ability, despite her own personal challenges, to continuously empower and encourage her daughter. This is a truly humanizing narrative of courage."

—Staci L. Dooney, M.ED, LMHC, LLC

"The story itself is beautiful and simple, but its simplicity is exactly what makes it so captivating. A masterful work."

—Kevin Penwell
President, Tucket Publishing

This book is dedicated to my mum, Marian F. Ciampa.
My friend and angel.

Your light will never fade.

Shine on.

Table of Contents

Foreword

How do you thank someone for giving you the gift of life? Not just life in the sense of existence; life in the sense of essence, spirit, vitality and soul. And how do you thank them, if they are no longer here? This had been my dilemma for several years: wanting more than anything to thank the woman who shaped my life in more ways than could be counted. It seemed as though the yearning to express my gratitude multiplied with each year that passed. At the same time, as days went by, I realized this longing was my inner need for certainty: Did she really know how much I loved her? How much I missed her? How thankful I was for everything she did for me? Did she know how much of an inspiration she was to me...and still is?

January 2007 marked the fourteenth anniversary of my mother's death. The occasion was especially difficult because it represented her absence for over half of my life. She died when

I was fourteen years old, which meant that she had now been gone equally as long as I had her. I also realized that if I measured my own years in the length of my mother's, that my life would be halfway over. Needless to say, a day which never came easily, was extraordinarily disheartening that particular year. To lift my spirits, I decided to treat the event as the fourteenth anniversary of my mum's *life*. After all, that's what anniversaries are for, right….celebration? In Ireland, where my mother's family was from, a traditional Irish wake was more of a party than a funeral. It consisted of the gathering of family and friends, plenty of food and drink to intoxicate the senses, and the absolute revelry of the departed person's life. Not a time for tears, it was the traditional Irish way of celebrating one's life and ensuring a good send off. Although this tradition was not as common as it once was, I decided to revive its philosophy for myself. At least for a day.

I began to write about one of my favorite subjects, my mum. She always had a way of exhilarating people, and clearly hadn't lost her touch. My few hours of writing that day turned into days and months, over which I released practically every emotion I'd ever held. I laughed and cried, realized and wondered, reminisced and imagined, and in doing so I had an epiphany. While writing, I started to think about how many people had come in and out of this world, who had led equally as magnificent and courageous lives as my mother, yet were known only by those who experienced them personally. How many great stories could be told if we could only learn of them? How many souls could be impacted and touched forever, if only the extraordinary lives of ordinary people were accounted for?

For these reasons, I decided to share my mother with the world. I chose to expose all sides of her life, as her humanity was defined by her strengths as well as her weaknesses. Mum was the genuine article, as human as they come. She was anything but ordinary. I think you will find her as familiar as your very best friend, and as courageous as your most well-loved hero. In this memoir, I hope to convey her spirit and attitude, as they embody what I believe to be essential determinants in understanding this enigma we know as life, and finding happiness within it. This book is a tribute to her life, her influence, and her passion.

Melinda Ferreira

Hello My Friend
I See You There
Just As You Said You'd Be
I Hear Your Laugh And See Your Smile
It's Good To Be With You For A While
Just The Two of Us
In This Place
I Feel Your Grace
Shining Down This Day
They Say I'm The Image of You Now
Can You See The Resemblance?
I Hope You're Proud
I Hope You Can See
Who I've Become, Who I Still Want To Be
My Mother's Daughter
Clearly
To Be Half The Woman
With Half The Strength
To Measure This Life
Not In Its Length
But In Moments Shared With Those I Love
To Always Wave To My Angels Above
To Live
To Laugh
To Love
To Share
I Realize When My Time Ends Here
The Light You Shine Will Draw Me Near
Rays Of Grace
In The Sky
Shine Over Me
Until I Die
Evolve Me
And Open My Eyes
So Once Again I Can See
The Beautiful Woman
Who Gave Life To Me

CHAPTER 1

Angels

Unexpected moments of grace are often bestowed upon us by angels attempting to awaken our souls. Some of the most monumental events in our lives take place in the most ordinary of circumstances, when we are least expectant. For me, a simple car ride with my mother, on a beautiful fall New England afternoon, was one of those occasions. Not until years later would I fully comprehend how deeply this journey would affect my life. Not that the experience didn't have an impact on me when it occurred, but as with many childhood experiences, my capacity to absorb the full magnitude of the situation was not fully developed. Nevertheless, seeing angels for the first time, at the tender age of eight, was pretty damn amazing. And who better than my mum, to introduce me to them.

It was an absolutely perfect autumn day in Massachusetts. The smell in the air, saturated with the aroma of crisp leaves and wood burning fires, was simply intoxicating. The colors of the sky were far more brilliant than in other seasons, with countless shades of reds and purples mesmerizing the dusk. A pure indulgence of the senses, this had always been my favorite time of year. My mother and I were returning home from Holbrook after having taken my grandmother to Mass. Atypical of most children, this ritual was one of my favorite pastimes. I was always filled with a sense of happiness and peace when accompanied by these two women. As they were capable of doing in any setting, they made the environment of church one in which I felt authentically at home. No pressure. No guilt. No memorization. Just togetherness. Pulling away from Grammy's house, we looked back to see her, as always, sitting at the kitchen window waving and blowing kisses to us until we were out of sight. This was her hallmark, and one of my favorite things in life. I remember asking my mum if Gram had always been so loving and gentle. I'd never met anyone as kind and good-natured. "She's always been my angel, Melin, and my best friend." I'd never heard of a person referred to as an angel before. It didn't make sense to me. Angels were with God. They were in the sky, with wings and halos. When I asked for clarification, my mother explained, "God sends angels in many forms, Sweetie. They are as present here on earth as they are in Heaven. This may be difficult for you to understand, but people can be angels. Some of your angels are present in your life right now. You just might not recognize them as such because their purpose in your existence may not yet be apparent. There are also those angels who have yet to come into your world, but they will, and in doing so they will open your eyes to beauty." Clearly seeing my confusion, she tried to clarify. "Not everything is as you read Sweetheart," she said. "Certain things are factual, and other things are meant to be a guide for you to follow and interpret. Remember, there's no one way of looking at anything.

You never have to accept anything as it is given to you. Always imagine. Always think. There are certain things that exist and are true whether people believe in them or not. Believe me, Melin, angels do exist. The question is whether or not we can recognize them when they walk into our lives." While this conversation could have been dramatically incomprehensible, my mother had an amazing talent of explaining things in a way which made perfect sense to me. She had a way with words. Every story, every explanation, every memory....was better told when my mum was the narrator. She made everything seem beautiful.

We continued our chat about angels as we turned onto a small stretch of highway which connected Avon to my hometown of Stoughton, Massachusetts, a midsized community about thirty minutes south of Boston. When my mother stopped her story mid-sentence, I looked over to see her grinning. She was clearly amused. Her smirk was not the kind that resulted from seeing something comical. She was instead smiling as if she'd just spotted an old friend from afar, and saw that he or she was up to the same old tricks. She had the look of relieved happiness of one who realized that a dear friend, despite time and distance, had not changed. In fact they were exactly as she remembered. This knowing, sentimental gaze in Mum's eyes prompted me to follow their fixedness toward the horizon, where I saw what seemed like hundreds of beams of light pouring through the soft autumn clouds. I'd always been fond of this display of nature, and held it as one of the more marvelous sights on earth. There had always been something wondrous about it. As only she could do, Mum succeeded in taking something beautiful and elevating it into something absolutely breathtaking.

"What are you smiling at?" I asked her. She pointed at the exquisite display of light in front of us. "You see those beams of light coming through the clouds?" As I looked up to the sky, there now seemed to be even more rays shining through. At least a million, was my safe estimate. Gently, Mum put her hand to her lips, blew a kiss toward the gorgeous spectacle, then turned her hand outward and waved. "Every time you see that, Sweetheart, when you see those rays of light coming through the clouds, wave to them. Those are your angels waving down to you from Heaven." For a moment, I stopped breathing. My jaw physically dropped and my normally squinty little blue eyes widened with pure awe. I felt as if I'd been let in on the greatest secret, the greatest revelation in the history of the world. Mum had just introduced me to my angels. It made perfect sense, yet I never would have come to this realization unless she had shared it with me. There they were, literally shining down on me from the sky. The sight instantly took on an entirely new meaning of beauty for me, incomparable to anything I could have possibly imagined. Thanks to Mum, I now had a direct contact with Heaven. A tangible, visible connection. Immediately, I began to think of how many times I had previously seen this beautiful vision and not realized its significance. For the first time in my young life, I realized how much I didn't know. Of what else was I not yet aware? By what other wonders was I surrounded that I hadn't yet discovered? My mind was racing with blissful amazement. I felt enormously small, as I had just encountered a new and fundamental conception in life. My hands were far from being wrapped around this new reality, but one thing was for certain. There was something else out there, something much bigger than me. I could feel it in my bones as I looked at my new friends in the sky. While I couldn't pinpoint it, I knew that it was something more quietly powerful than anything I'd ever known; something infinitely present. My little body filled with glorious wonderment. Never had revelation of unconsciousness been so invigorating. And never had something felt so real to me. This was my first recognition of blessedness.

Chapter 2

The Laugh

THE EARLIEST MEMORY I HAVE OF MY MOTHER IS OF HER LAUGH. WHEN I stretch my mind to recall the first stages of my childhood, I remember knowing this before even knowing her face. That irresistible, from-the-depths-of-your-soul laugh. My father told me that the first time I ever smiled was in response to my mother's laughter. I don't doubt it for a second. Mum laughed harder and more often than perhaps any human being in recorded history. Hers was the kind of belly laugh that was completely genuine and uninhibited. When it got a hold of her, my mother would literally lose her breath for several seconds at a time, and then burst into short-winded cackles which typically sent everyone in her vicinity into hysterics. She was contagious, in every sense of the word.

Mum was the quintessential life of the party, and people loved being around her. She was everyone's favorite everything: daughter, sister, aunt, cousin, friend, you name it. My mother was adored by a wide range of people. Regardless of age, background, temperament, or profession, Mum could charm anyone. She possessed a unique authenticity which made everyone around her feel comfortable. People always listened when she spoke. Whether it was her natural storytelling ability, legendary sense of humor, sheer beauty, or perhaps a combination of all these things that unfailingly captivated those around her, it was magical to watch. She was naturally beautiful, with long brown hair and slate blue eyes that disappeared into slits when she laughed or smiled, which was most of the time. High, rosy cheek bones accented her face, with a pointy little nose and thin lips completing her appearance. More times than I can recall, people commented that she had the map of Ireland on her face. Though I didn't understand the expression, I developed an immediate affection for it, as my mother was the most beautiful woman in the world to me.

Beyond physical attractiveness and comic relief, what made my mother truly magnetic was her capacity to connect with others. An amazing listener, Mum was inherently nonjudgmental, and emitted an unspoken understanding of acceptance to those who confided in her. She was the ultimate confidant, possessing a level of depth and concern most find only in a spouse or parent. No matter the given situation, Mum knew how to react. She was blessed with the rare and vital ability to comprehend the legitimate needs of others, and knew when to give advice and when to just listen. This awareness is what made her so extraordinary, and it caused nearly everyone who ever met my mother to fall in love with her. I've never heard so many different people refer to one individual as their best friend; a true testament to a life well lived. Her name was Marian Ciampa, and I am proud to say, that she was also *my* best friend.

CHAPTER 3

The Fam

ONE OF THE SUREST WAYS OF GAINING A BETTER UNDERSTANDING OF A person is by taking a look at her family. My mother's family, both the one into which she was born, as well as that which she established with my father, was her life.

Marian Frances Lynch took her first breath on June 27, 1948. She was the youngest of seven children born to Mary and Matthew Lynch, who had emigrated from Ireland to Boston in the 1920's. My grandfather moved the family from Jamaica Plain to Holbrook, Massachusetts in the mid 1950's, into a home he built with his own hands. Like many Irish-American families at the time, they worked hard and lived humbly. As I understand it, my mum was the consummate baby of the bunch, seeking mischievousness anywhere it could be found. Either as a result of being born later in my grandparents lives (Pa was forty-four and Grammy was thirty-six at the time of her birth), or perhaps utilizing the same innate charm she would use to enchant people throughout her life, my mother got away with a hell of a lot more than did her older brothers and sisters, from what I've been told. No surprise there. My grandmother used to tell me that Mum would get into more mischief, yet less trouble or consequence, than anyone she ever knew. She said it was hard for anyone, including my grandfather, who had a wicked temper in his day, to be angry or stay angry at my mother if she did something wrong. "She could always make you laugh," Grammy would say. "No matter how intense or grim the situation, Marian had a way of breaking you down and making you laugh. It was maddening and wonderful at the same time. You'd get a little miffed because you knew she'd gotten you, but in the same right you were glad she did. Marian was always a little ray of sunshine."

On July 5, 1969, Mum cast her radiance into the life of a twenty-year-old kid from Saugus named Jim Ciampa, my father. Dad said when he met my mother he thought he was looking at a brunette Ann Margret. It was instant chemistry. They married three years later and had my older brother Jimmy in September of 1976. I followed two years after, and my younger brother Matt completed the family eighteen months later. I was daddy's little girl from day one. Some of my first memories, from around the age of three, are of getting into my signature Dr. Denton pajamas and hopping into my father's lap to watch Red Sox games on our living room television. He taught me everything about the game of baseball, which became the second love in my life. He was the first. I simply idolized my father. He was larger than life to me. The prototypical Italian-Irish American, Dad has always been very loud and very proud. You can typically hear my father coming before you can see him. He was every bit as much the life of the party as my mother, which made for some famous bashes at our house when we were little. He's always been handsome, sporting a premature silver head of hair which he and my mother sadly attempted to dye one night before leaving for a Disney vacation. Needless to say, pool chlorine and bad hair dye don't mix well together, so my father spent the rest of the trip wearing a baseball cap to cover up his green locks. Lesson learned. Besides that one botched effort for the fountain of youth, Dad has had no reason to attempt to look younger. Pound for pound, he is quite possibly the strongest person I've ever met. The self-proclaimed "Worm Man" has been wholesaling fishing bait in New England for over forty years. That amount of time spent loading and unloading tons of bait on and off of his truck has kept him in strapping shape. Small in stature, my father stands about 5'8" tall on his best day, although his pride and his license will tell you that he is 5'9 and 3/4". Over the years, we've all just learned to nod and smile at this enigma. The one thing we never wanted to do was make Jim Ciampa angry. His temper could accurately be compared to that of Dr. David Banner when he transformed into the Incredible Hulk. Somehow my brothers and I, whether intentionally or not, never failed to ignite it.

Jimbo is my older brother, and one of the smartest people I know. He's one of those individuals who can read a textbook on microbiology and recite it back to you an hour later, with full comprehension. When we were kids he used to ask for microscopes and books for Christmas, as opposed to toys or typical gifts. Beyond his natural brilliance, he has always been a very peaceful person. I don't have many memories of just him and me as siblings before my brother Matt arrived, but from what I'm told he was very happy when I was born. He was good to me and liked having a friend, whereas many children become jealous and territorial when someone else comes along and steals their thunder. His reaction to me is very indicative of the benevolence he's displayed throughout his life.

Matt's arrival was a very different story. Born nearly two months premature, he weighed only three pounds at birth. The complications of his delivery nearly ended both his and my mother's lives, yet they both survived. I believe this experience bonded them intensely, as they shared a special kinship throughout life that was uniquely theirs. Eventually Matt put on enough weight for Jimmy and me to use him as our personal guinea pig. Though my older brother was reluctant, I eventually corrupted him into helping me with several "experiments," which included boxing Matt in a storage container and pushing him down the stairs, feeding him urine-laden Cheeseballs, and swinging him so hard in his bouncy chair that he actually did a full three-hundred and sixty degree rotation. No matter what we did to him, my baby brother would laugh his little heart out. Though I was initially skeptical of this little man who had taken my parents' attention away from me, I was helplessly overcome by his lovable demeanor. My wariness quickly converted into an unconditional adoration, which remains to this day.

In true Leo fashion, I've saved myself for last. Much like Mum and Dad, I have always been extremely extroverted. Never failing to miss an opportunity to be the center of attention, I began playing sports practically before I could walk. I fantasized about becoming the first professional woman baseball player, and starting at shortstop for the Sox. Quickly, I developed into the world's biggest tomboy. My haircut was typically as short as either of my brothers', I refused to wear dresses, and I even tried several times to urinate while standing upright. After a few failed attempts and the disgusting feeling of my stream running down my legs, I gave up on the peeing thing. Needless to say, I made things interesting. One year, the night before Easter Sunday, I thought it was a good idea to cut my own hair. No more than five or six years old at the time, I decided it was far too long for the latest career I had in mind. Using a pair of construction scissors, I hid inside my closet and chopped my golden locks nearly down to my scalp. Mission accomplished, I proudly strolled into the kitchen to show Mum my new do. From her deer-in-the-headlights stare, it was clear to me that she thought it was as awesome as I did. She walked toward me, took the scissors out of my hands, and placed them on the counter. She then ran her hand gently over my head and what remained of my hair. Looking up at her, I said, "Do you like it Mummy?" She took my face in both of her hands. "What did you do, Sweetheart?" With pure excitement I explained the basis of my decision. "I'm gonna be an astronaut. So I needed to cut my hair so my head can fit in my helmet." As profound as I thought it was, my rationale sent my mother into one of her greatest belly laughs of all time. Mum's laughter was by far the funniest thing on earth to me, so even though I couldn't possibly make sense of her amusement, her cackling caused me to go into hysterics with her. We ended up in convulsions on the kitchen floor. "You're an astronaut Melin, that is for sure." When we finally caught our breath, she sat me down at the table. "I'm not angry at you Sweetie, but you could have really hurt yourself with those big scissors," she said. "I'll tell you what, from now on if you ever want a haircut, whether for your space helmet or your Red Sox helmet, I'll either do it for you or take you to get one. Deal?" Thinking her offer was pretty fair, I nodded in agreement. Unfortunately, the other half of her bargain required me to wear a bonnet for Easter the next day. When I opened my mouth to argue this point, Mum gave me a look that silently told me to stop while I was ahead, so I did. Very rarely did her normally light-hearted nature expose its sternness, but when it did, I knew better than to challenge it. Then using a smaller set of clippers, she did the best she could to fix the atrocity I had created on my head. To be honest, it didn't turn out so badly. At the very least, it looked a hell of a lot better than my original masterpiece. Easter went off without a hitch, and thanks to Mum's strategic wardrobe selection for me, no one noticed the defective trim. The experience, however, had lasting effects. I'm pretty sure I'm the only person in the world who views Easter bonnets as "mea culpa."

CHAPTER 4

Lesson #1

ONE OF THE GREATEST PARTS OF GROWING UP AS A TOMBOY WAS THAT my mother never pressured me to be something I wasn't. She would occasionally ask me if I wanted to wear more feminine outfits, or if I wanted her to put barrettes in my hair. When I said no, that was the end of it. No pressure and no judgment.

There was one female relative in particular who used to loathe the fact that I behaved boyishly. During one of the holidays, she confronted my mother in front of me. "Marian, if you don't stop dressing her like that she's going to turn out to be a dyke!" This woman, while famous for expressing her opinions, often times without regard, had crossed the line. Overhearing the comment, I didn't understand what her apparent accusation even meant, but her tone was laden with disgust, which left me inexplicably ashamed. I felt awful about myself, and didn't understand why. As my face flushed with embarrassment, I began to well up. Lifting my chin with her hand, Mum raised my watery eyes up to hers. They looked straight into me, and were intense with love. She slowly shook her head from left to right, implicitly telling me not to cry. Desperately, I fought back the tears. Calmly, she turned to my critic and said, "She's my daughter, and as long as she's happy, that's all that will ever matter to me." The teardrops my mother had just motioned me to resist now streamed down my face, but with a completely different sentiment than that with which they were created. For the first time in my life, I cried out of pure joy. It is difficult for me to quantify the importance of this moment. In one encounter, I was introduced to the concepts of self-consciousness and self-esteem. Having now irreversibly learned of the former, the latter would become instrumental in shaping my character. My mother's reassuring words in this instance proved to be the root of my dignity. Not only did she teach me to be happy with myself, and true to myself, she also taught me to respect myself. "No one can make you feel inferior without your consent." Mum loved quotes, and she shared this one from Eleanor Roosevelt with me as she wiped the tears from my face. I never felt so loved.

CHAPTER 5

The Age of Innocence

FOR THE AVERAGE PERSON, IT IS DIFFICULT TO IMAGINE BEING TRULY carefree. Perhaps only when we strain to remember the early stages of childhood, for a time of pure naïveté and happiness, can we grasp this concept. Our daily responsibilities and distractions can easily jade our recollections of such times, lending to perceptions of reality based solely in the present. Some people intentionally forget the past because of an inability to deal with the disconnect between the light-heartedness that once was and the discontent which currently exists. Sometimes the sheer examination of one's life and measurement of personal satisfaction can be painful, especially if the introspection reveals shortcomings and unfulfillment. For others, however, the recollection of childhood bliss provides purification, and reminds them of an innocence that still exists in the world. I am one of the lucky ones who can reminisce to a time of complete joy, when I truly had not a care in the world, and thank God for those occasions. My upbringing was by no means perfect. It was filled with both wonderful and painful memories, but so life unfolds. Nothing is without its flaws. In the grand scale of things, however, measuring both the good and the bad, I am blessed to have the former far outweigh the latter. Over the years, focusing on and being thankful for this one point has made a dramatic impact on my happiness.

Some of the fondest memories of my life are from childhood. Every year, we spent practically half the summer down the Cape (that's Cape Cod to the non-Bostonian). As mentioned, my father ran his own company wholesaling fishing bait, which was a seasonal business that began in early spring and lasted through the end of October, the most fruitful and popular fishing months in New England. Most of his customers were in southern Massachusetts, Rhode Island, and Cape Cod. Because his busiest time of the year was when my brothers and I were on school vacation, we didn't get to spend much time with him over the summer. So he would rent a cottage and arrange for my mother to take us down the Cape for a few weeks, where it was easy for him to visit us because he typically ended his route there.

We spent our mornings eating Mum's famous scrambled eggs and ham, listening to her Elvis tapes, and packing coolers with sandwiches and chips to take to the beach. My mother was a beach junkie. She absolutely adored the ocean. It was in her blood. And thanks to her, it's in mine and my brothers' as well. Mum wasn't necessarily a sun worshipper, although she used to tan impressively for an Irishman. What she really loved were the natural elements of this atmosphere—the smell of the salt water, the sound of the surf crashing on shore, the sight of the sun glistening on the ocean, the touch of warm sand on her feet, and the taste of summer on her lips. This was her Utopia. It didn't get much better. While Jimmy, Matt and I spent countless hours making sandcastles, catching jellyfish with our nets, and playing stickball, Marian would be reading one of her books. The woman read more than anyone I've ever known, which undoubtedly satiated her love of words and fostered her talent with them. I never paid much attention to what she read, but if we needed to, my brothers and I were highly skilled at getting our mother to take her focus off her hobby. Thanks to a certain classic Alfred Hitchcock movie, Mum was terrified (not frightened, but *terrified*) of birds, especially seagulls. She hated them with the fire of a thousand suns, and fondly referred to them as "rats with wings." Fully aware of this disdain, my brothers and I would strategically sit and eat our lunches about five feet behind my mother's beach chair. Realizing that seagulls are scavengers, we would break our sandwich bread into tiny pieces and throw them in Mum's direction, preferably just behind her so she couldn't see what we were doing. Like clockwork, a shower of seagulls would dive at our mother's chair, desperately fighting for the morsels we had tossed at her. In a panic, she would flail her arms and swing her book to disperse them, but still managed to come up with some of the most creative cursing I've ever heard. I never realized birds could be "whoremasters," or furthermore, could be threatened to have their "balls cut off." Who even knew they had balls? Anyway, these fight-or-flight fits used to send me and my brothers into utter hysteria, which unfailingly blew our cover. While we endured short but well deserved reprimandings, we had to struggle to suppress our laughter. Though this would initially piss her off even further, Mum always seemed to end up giggling with us. We eventually had to develop different strategies for this pastime (which never seemed to get old): including incremental bread tossing, which allowed the birds more time to gather in between tosses; "playing dead" (aka pretending we were asleep on our towels) immediately after throwing food in Mum's direction, which would leave her wondering if her dive-bombing friends were simply an inconvenient coincidence; and then of course, the fake injury. This tactic was a collective effort and worked like a charm. One of us would fake impairment in order to lure my mother away from her book. Then, once she wasn't looking, the remaining two kids would dump chips all over her folding chair, creating a bombardment of beach birds that would decidedly desecrate her space. I'd like to say we knew when to say when, but some things just don't lose their humor. Every once in a while, we'd get a little whack on the backside for our actions, but it was well worth it. While we drove her nuts with our antics, I think Mum found our methods fairly impressive.

Memories such as these provide me with constant reminders of the humor and innocence that filled my childhood. In many ways, I lived a very normal and happy youth. There were certain realities and circumstances, however, which juxtaposed the simplicity of those years.

Chapter 6

Blissful Ignorance

IGNORANCE IS BLISS. THAT IS, IF ONE'S UNAWARENESS SHELTERS HER FROM knowledge that could irreversibly change her life in a negative way. For a good part of my childhood, I lived as most other children do: in my own world. I spent my time playing with my brothers, dreaming of becoming a professional athlete, and worrying about nothing. I had no sense of time, vanity, calories, money, political correctness, or drama between friends. The guide to my life was simple: be a good girl, be happy, and don't hurt anyone. For all the rules I was given as a child, these were the standards instilled by my parents. For the most part, I think I followed them pretty well.

Despite the simplicity that defined this part of my life, there were intricacies woven into it which exposed me to sobering and undeniable realities. As I mentioned, my parents were known for throwing amazing parties, sometimes quite spontaneously. That being said, the liquor cabinet in our house was always stocked, and I was surrounded by alcohol from a very early age. When I was a toddler, I recognized smells more than anything. Scotch. Whiskey. Beer. Vodka. Ironically, I was never really tempted to sneak any of these spirits because their aromas turned my stomach. Besides, I didn't know any better. Because I had no comprehension of the potential "perks" of liquor, drinking did not appeal to me. I made absolutely no association between behavior and alcohol. The very concept wouldn't have even made sense to me. Nonetheless, booze was as normal and permanent a fixture in our home as groceries or milk.

As years went by, I naturally took more interest in my parents' parties. This is perhaps when I developed my infamous "FOMS:" Fear Of Missing Something. I've always had a desire to be in the middle of the action. The house in which we lived was perfect for entertaining, complete with an inground pool, a huge yard, a massive kitchen and sunroom. The air was constantly filled with music and laughter, two of my favorite things. How could I possibly stay away? Typically, we kids would swim in the pool and play in the back yard during the day, and then go inside to watch movies and play games until we eventually fell asleep. As my desire to be part of the fun increased, I would force myself to stay awake after the other children had gone to bed. I'd then sneak out of my bedroom and rejoin the festivities. Most of the time, my parents marched me straight back to bed as soon as they learned of my antics. On a few occasions, however, they would let me stay up and hang to a reasonable degree. Even though my involvement was typically limited to watching TV in the next room, I felt honored to be part of the excitement, which always seemed to increase with night's progression.

The notion of drunkenness did not come to me in an isolated or definitive moment. Instead it was a gradual, nameless familiarity. When people think of the stereotypical symptoms of intoxication, the things that most likely come to mind are slurred speech, staggered walking, incomprehension, inebriation. Most of us can immediately recognize these characteristics at face value. A seven year old, on the other hand, probably cannot. She can, however, sense that something is off when she sees it with her own eyes. A subtle but uncomfortable confusion sets in, and she realizes something is wrong…yet she can't pinpoint it. This is how *I* felt, anyway, in witnessing varying degrees of alcoholism in my home. Parties were one thing—even as a little girl, I understood that there was a certain atmosphere that surrounded parties that wasn't part of the daily routine. Quite frankly, I couldn't get enough of it. My greatest joy in life has always been the company of my family and friends. What began to unsettle me, however, was seeing Mum in the same state of insobriety (or worse) when no one was around. Of course at the time I didn't recognize her actions for what they were. When she slurred her speech, I honestly thought it was because she was tired. When she stumbled, I thought she was sick. Throughout my childhood, my mother was in and out of hospitals constantly, for a variety of reasons. High blood pressure. Colitis. Strokes. I swear the woman was plagued with health issues her entire life. Consequently, I mistook many of her drunken episodes for illness. And I was positive that the countless medications she took for her ailments were responsible for her grogginess. The truth is I probably would have never comprehended my mother's alcoholism, or its extent, had it not been for my father's exposure of it.

For as much and as madly as they loved one another, my mum and dad fought more than any other couple I've known. In hindsight, it makes perfect sense to me since they were two of the most stubborn, most strongly opinionated people to have dared enter into marriage together. My father was perhaps a bit more bull-headed than my mother, but she never conceded to him if they didn't see eye to eye. Dad has always held a "my way or the highway" attitude, which never meshed well with my mum's rebellious nature. Hence, the combination of his inflexibility and her unyieldingness made for a very hostile environment at times. Many times, actually. There is one specific argument, however, which changed my life and how I viewed everything in it forever. Once again, ignorance is bliss.

Chapter 7

Naïveté Lost

ONE OF THE GREATEST JOYS IN MY YOUNG LIFE WAS SPORTS, ESPECIALLY softball. The town of Stoughton, Massachusetts was well known in the area for breeding outstanding athletes in this particular arena. Although I had a talent for the game, the girls with whom I played were simply phenomenal. No matter which age division I was involved with, I was quite often the youngest one on the team. By playing with older and superior athletes, I was able to take full advantage of their extra training and develop my own skill set to a similar level.

From the very first time I stepped onto the field, my parents were my biggest fans. No matter how farfetched or lofty my goals, Mum would indulge in them with me. Her support was unwavering. Even though she never played herself, she adopted my passion as her own; one of the many things which made her an incredible mother. She never missed a game. Dad spent every spare minute he had after work practicing with me in the front yard. Regardless of his schedule, he would somehow manage to see me play, even if he showed up in the last inning. On one particular August afternoon, I had a game at a nearby school in my hometown. I was about nine or ten years old at the time. As always, Mum drove me to the field and read her book while we were warming up. About an inning into the game, my father showed up, having come straight from work. I don't remember seeing my mother leave, but I noticed it when I got on base, looked over to see my "cheering section," and saw only my dad. I really didn't think much of it, as Mum could very well have just stepped away to the concession stand or bathroom. Or she could have made a quick trip home to do an errand, as she often did. I do remember, however, seeing the police show up at the field a few innings later. My team was batting, and I was sitting in the dugout, across from where my father was standing to watch the game. When the policeman first showed up, it looked like he was asking around to find someone. When he finally reached my father, I knew something was wrong. I was too far away to hear their conversation, but the fear I saw in Dad's eyes in response to what he was being told made my heart stop. My mind raced. I didn't know what to think. Was he was getting arrested for something? Did something happen to one of my brothers? Almost immediately, my father walked over to me and told me he had to go, and that I needed to get a ride home with one of the girls. Panicking, I asked what was wrong, but he had already started to walk away. As he rushed back towards the cop, he stopped to ask my friend's mother if she could give me a ride home. "There's been an emergency," I heard him say. My heart went from not beating to pounding out of my chest. In all the chaos, I had lost track of everything going on around me. "Come on, Melin… you're up!" yelled my coach from across the field. Somewhat dazed, I grabbed a bat and ran up to the plate. As I dug in, the umpire called time and asked me to turn around. He tapped his head, which was his way of telling me I had forgotten my helmet. Mortified, I ran back to the dugout to grab one, only to hear my hot-tempered manager scream at the top of his lungs, "Ciampa, get your head in the game!!!" I couldn't have been further away from that game if I tried. All I could see was my father getting into his truck and following the police cruiser out of the parking lot. My eyes started to fill. As I stepped into the batter's box, I remember thinking, "Don't cry. Don't make a scene." The lump in my throat made it difficult to breathe or swallow, and my vision was blurred by my tears. I struck out on three pitches.

When I finally made it home, I walked into a shouting match between my parents; one of the worst ever. Although I didn't understand much of what was said, I did manage to grasp that Mum had been in a car accident. For the life of me, I couldn't understand, then, why my father was angry with her. He just kept yelling. "This has to stop." "You need to get help." "You were lucky this time." Confused, and upset with my father for being so mean to her, I walked toward my mother to give her a hug. I smelled the alcohol before I reached her. It wasn't an unfamiliar scent, just heavier than normal. She began to cry, and then stumbled as I embraced her, which enraged Dad even more. The fight escalated, with my father reprimanding my mother and her vehemently denying his accusations. Finally I broke in, "Why are you mad at her? She could have died!" Nearing his breaking point, my father paused, as if carefully contemplating his choice of words. "That's exactly why I'm mad at her," he said. My mother retorted. "You're no saint," she slurred. "Don't you dare make me out to be the bad guy in front of my daughter." Now even more baffled, I started arguing with Dad. "Why don't you leave her alone. She's sick and she's tired and the last thing she needs right now is you yelling at her!" Then he snapped. "She's not tired…she's drunk. And she almost killed herself this afternoon by driving the car into a frigging stone wall." Suddenly there was silence. I went numb. It was the first time I had ever heard of my mother doing something bad. I couldn't look at her, as if I would see another person if I did. For the first time, the possibility dawned on me that this distinct smell, the slurred speech, the staggered walk…was not what I had believed it to be…that it could be something else entirely. A million thoughts raced through my mind. Did this mean every time she momentarily disappeared from a game that she was sneaking off to drink? No…I refused to believe it. Maybe just this once. "Why are you doing this to me?" she said to him, weeping now. Her words were almost incomprehensible. "I was just tired. This is your fault." I didn't know whom to believe, but it didn't matter. Instinctively, I sided with Mum, purely because it broke my heart to see her crying. The damage had been done though. As much as I wanted to block out what my father had said, I couldn't. This revelation was permanent, and immeasurably hurtful. It caused a disheartening domino effect, unintentionally eliciting multiple realizations. Overwhelmed and not knowing what to say or do, I did the only thing I could think of. I started to walk my mother upstairs, so she could rest. She stumbled again at the base of the staircase, and a third time before we reached the top, landing hard on the steps. I was scared, and didn't want my father to hear us out of fear that he would start yelling again. Putting her arm around my shoulder, I attempted to lift her. She was deadweight. Before I could react, I felt Dad kneel down by my side. "I've got her, Melin." He slipped his arms underneath her back and her legs, lifted her up, and carried her into their bedroom. Laying Mum down gently on the bed, he sat next to her. She was completely unconscious. For several moments my father remained motionless, staring at my mother. I couldn't see his face, as he had his back to me. Although I'd never seen him cry, I felt as if he may have been at that moment. It seemed as if he was completely unaware that I was still standing there. After a deep breath, he untied and removed Mum's shoes, then pulled up the sheets and comforter to cover her. Finally, he gently brushed her face and hair with his hand, and kissed her on the forehead. I heard him whisper, "I love you, Monk" as he pulled away. His voice cracked with emotion. "Monk," short for monkey, was their term of endearment for one another. As Dad stood up to leave the room, he suddenly realized I had been watching him. He froze for an instant, a look of guilt on his face. His eyes were filled with tears. Clearly he realized the impact of what I'd seen and heard. It was as if he had told me that Santa Claus wasn't real. He closed the bedroom door behind him and took my face in his hands. "Everything's gonna be alright Pumpkin," he said. "Mummy's sick. Not the way you thought, but she's still sick. And we're going to get her help." I thought I understood what he was saying. I felt so bad for Mum…I'd never known anyone as sick as she. Yet the realization started to set in. Things were not as I had once known. The magic of Christmas morning is never quite the same for a child who no longer believes.

CHAPTER 8

Cloudy Skies

THE NEXT FEW YEARS WERE TUMULTUOUS TO SAY THE LEAST. MUM'S drinking continued, despite several efforts on both my parents' parts to help her stop. It came in waves, it seemed. Sometimes several months would go by with no alcohol-related incidents. It appeared that the AA meetings and the counseling sessions which she and my father attended together were working. I eventually realized, however, that my mother's sickness had not gone away at all. It had been temporarily pacified by therapy, but the underlying addiction had not been treated. Her binges had merely been kept well hidden.

Sunday night was Chinese food night in my house. It was a treasured family ritual to me. Nothing like pork fried rice and chicken wings to end the weekend right! After one of my Sunday afternoon softball games, we all stopped home to freshen up before going out to eat. Ready within five minutes (more excited about my favorite food than what my hair looked like…again, the beauty of being a tomboy), I grabbed my favorite book and went downstairs to read for a few minutes while everyone else was getting ready. I sat in my father's chair, which was in the living room, next to the kitchen. Sitting back in it, I couldn't see into the next room. A few pages in to my novel, I heard something that resembled glass clanging. Although sure that I was the only one downstairs at the time, I leaned forward to peek inside the kitchen. Seeing no one, I chalked it up to things maybe shifting around in the dishwasher and went back to reading my book. About thirty seconds went by and I heard the noise again, this time accompanied by the faint sound of movement on the floor. With my curiosity now peaked, I quietly stood up from Dad's chair and walked, as if on eggshells, into the kitchen to investigate. Again, I saw an empty kitchen. Or so I thought. Our kitchen was fairly large, with a unique layout. When entering from the living room, the table at which we ate was on the left, and beyond it was a wrap around peninsula with bar stools. So for all intents and purposes, anything below countertop level inside the area surrounded by the peninsula would go unseen, unless one was close enough to see over the counter and into that space. For some reason I started to get nervous. The sounds I heard were not clear, but rather muffled. I thought it must have been one of our cats playing with something on the ground. To my dismay and shock, I was wrong. Walking farther into the kitchen, I was stopped in my tracks when I saw a hand rise into the air from behind the counter. Someone was on the floor. I took two more tip-toed steps forward. When the figure came into sight it took my breath away. I took a quick gasp in and then stopped breathing completely, not wanting to be noticed. I had definitely walked in on something I should not have. There, sprawled on the ground, was my mother, swigging Bacardi directly out of the bottle. Her eyes were half closed and half rolling into the back of her head. I was paralyzed with fear. Fear that she'd see me. Fear that Dad would walk in. Fear that she'd pass out again. Fear that she'd be upset with me when she realized that I knew she was still drinking. Almost immediately, I reversed my direction and headed back toward the parlor. I prayed she didn't notice me, as there was absolutely no way, on her end, of explaining what I'd seen. As I quietly lowered myself down into Dad's seat, I recalled the promises my mother had made. *No more drinking for Mummy. I don't need it anymore.* I'd been lied to, by the person I admired most in the world. How could she do this? To herself? To me and my brothers? To Dad? What could possibly be so great about drinking, that she would lower herself to secretly guzzling booze on the floor of our kitchen? Despite the countless drunken episodes I'd seen in my young life, this single incident defined alcoholism to me. It unveiled a side of my mother I'd never seen before; secretive, deceitful, out of control, helpless. Quite literally, it had brought her to her knees. Suddenly, I heard my father coming down the stairs. Once again, I started to experience that stomach-turning feeling of anxiety rise within me. I felt my face burn and my heart pound out of my chest. If he took the normal route into the kitchen, which would have been a left off the stairs, and through the dining room, he would walk directly into the scene I had just witnessed, as Mum would be positioned on the floor right in front of him. If I distracted him however, and called him into the parlor, maybe that would buy some time for my mother to gather herself. It was my only shot at this night not turning into a total and utter disaster. "Dad!" I yelled from his seat. I heard him change his route off the stairs and head in my direction. I flew out of his chair and met him at the entrance of the room, so we were not in view of the kitchen. "What?" he said. "Come look outside," I responded. It was all I could think of at the time. I didn't know what I was going to say once we arrived there, but I had to sidetrack him for at least a few more seconds. Opening the front door to a whole lot of nothing, my dad looked at me, confused. "What am I supposed to be looking at Melin?" Stumped, but determined to occupy him, I grabbed his hand and pulled him out onto the front steps. After a few moments of standing in silence (something my father cannot bear), he became annoyed. Realizing there was nothing worthy of sightseeing in the front yard, he turned to walk back into the house. "Come on Pumpkin, let's go eat." Desperate, I blurted out the first thing I could think of. "Those birds were just out here dive-bombing Pudgy again!" Pudgy was one of our two cats at the time. Pleasantly plump (as her name implies), and painfully slow in her saunter, she was a preferred target for a particular species of birds which nested in our neighborhood. They would routinely circle above her, as if stalking their prey, then dive at her, sometimes knocking her down in her tracks. This infuriated my father, who possessed an extraordinary affection for our pets, especially Pudge. A few times he went as far as firing rocks into the sky and terminating a few of the feathered hunters. So of course, the very mention of these birds immediately dragged him back outside. Unfortunately the horizon was as clear as a blank canvas; not a winged creature in sight. Just as I swore up and down to Dad that I'd seen the attacks, my favorite fat cat waddled up the stairs. While I was relieved and grateful at her timing, as she gave some sense of credibility to my story, I knew my time was up. Seeing she was alright, my father headed back inside. I followed hesitantly, hoping intensely that Mum had heard us and pulled herself together. As I entered the kitchen, I felt as if I was about to view a train wreck. My body was tightened with nervous anticipation, my head turned slightly to the side to avoid seeing the impending disaster straight on. I put my hand to my mouth as I always did when frightened, almost as a defense mechanism to keep myself from gasping or convulsing at what I was about to encounter. Suddenly I heard the tea kettle whistling. Turning the corner, I saw my mother at the stove, standing as steady and straight as a soldier, making a cup of tea. "You want a cup before we go, Monk?" she said to my father. "Sure, I'll take one to fly," he responded. I couldn't believe my eyes. Not two minutes had passed since I'd seen my mother writhing on the floor with a bottle to her lips, and now she seemed completely unfazed. As relieved as I was that Mum had managed to compose herself, I was consequently exposed to her incredible ability to hide her addiction and its symptoms. As our eyes met, she gave me a huge smile and said, "You ready for your favorite food, Sweetie?!" Still in disbelief, I responded with a simple, "Yup." I didn't know whether to laugh or cry. My anger toward her dishonesty was overpowered by my appreciation of her avoiding a potentially huge blow out with Dad. Regardless, I'd seen all I needed to see. Little by little, my innocence was slipping away…along with my trust. Jimmy and Matt came down shortly after and we went out for our weekly feast. Had it not been for my accidental discovery, that night would have been one of the most uneventful but pleasant evenings in quite some time.

However, Mum's drinking eventually caught up with her. The fighting between her and my father escalated; the arguments almost always being linked to her alcoholism. Looking back now as an adult, I realize her addiction was a crutch for many things with which she was unhappy in her life. Although she was married to the love of her life, her marriage to Dad was not perfect. At times, the similarities which brought them together also drove them apart. For all his good intentions, my father has been known to drive people to the edge of insanity. When Dad's in a zone, his Type A, obsessive-compulsive personality can make even the most laid back person feel like he is having a panic attack. I don't think he's ever meant to have this effect on people. Rather I think it's a result of his being one of the most anxious and restless people I've ever known, and his means of releasing his own tension succeeds in putting others in a similar state. Consequently, the combination of his intense demeanor and her unwillingness to submit to it, created a highly stressful environment which my mother tried to conceal. Alcohol, I've come to understand, was a key outlet she used to escape from various sources of distain. Mum never wanted to appear unhappy, as she was virtually the most easygoing person in the world to those who knew her. She loved this persona, and in some ways, I believe she felt obligated to project it, despite her true feelings. Hence, a cover up was needed. Unfortunately, this vice became a staple in her daily routine, and managed to control not only her life, but ours as well. And just when I thought I'd seen the worst of this addiction and its effect on my mother, a fateful event took place which would give ultimatum to her life as well as her marriage.

Sometimes it takes a near death experience to open one's eyes to the value of life. Mum's alcoholism reached its pinnacle on a very peaceful Tuesday evening in the fall of 1989. She'd been upstairs reading, as she often did at night. My brothers and I were in the family room watching television, while my father was in the cellar (his "office") doing paperwork. The evening was enjoyably dormant. Fixated on the movie we were watching, I didn't hear my mother come out of her room at the top of the stairs. All concentration was broken however, when I heard a horrifying, thunderous bang at the base of the staircase. Its impact literally shook the house to its foundation. Jimmy, Matt, and I flew up out of our seats to see what had caused the jolt. I could hear Dad racing up the basement stairs, shouting obscenities. "What the hell was that!?" He reached the scene just moments after we did. "Jesus Christ...Marian!!" he screamed in fear. Mum had fallen down the stairs and landed hard against the wall at the landing, her head twisted awkwardly toward her body. She wasn't moving. Dad repeatedly yelled her name, yet she was unresponsive. Frantically, he turned to me and my brothers. "Get me the phone...NOW!!!" I ran into the parlor, grabbed the portable phone, and raced it back to my father. He was panicking;

his fingers shook as he dialed. "Oh my God…Mum!" Matt said, as tears filled his daunted eyes. He was thinking what we all were. "Is she dead?" he asked in a desperate voice. Suddenly my father cried out. "I need an ambulance! Twenty Michael Lane. My wife has fallen down the stairs…she's not breathing…"

Mum was in the hospital for several days. Beyond the minor injuries she suffered from the fall, which resulted from an alcohol-induced blackout, my mother had also suffered a stroke. Although I didn't learn of them until years later, she experienced about four of these near fatal episodes throughout her life. When she was well enough to be counseled, her physicians were brutally honest with her. Her alcoholism, combined with a family history of high blood pressure and stroke, was a disastrous combination which could likely lead to more serious consequences. The doctors told her if she did not quit drinking that she would be at high risk of encountering further and more devastating events in the future. Now faced with the ultimatum of living alcohol-free or potential death or disability, Mum was finally convinced to enter a long-term rehabilitation facility.

She spent ten weeks in a private program in Newport, Rhode Island. Though I didn't quite understand *where* she'd gone, I knew she'd gone somewhere to get better. That Thanksgiving was the first holiday of my life not spent at Grammy's house. Instead, we packed up the car and drove to Newport. It was our only opportunity, throughout the duration of Mum's stay, to visit her. It was very strange to say the least. I barely comprehended the concept of rehabilitation, which I guess in a way was a blessing for me, and my mother. Because we only grasped the very surface of why she was there, my brothers and I didn't really talk about it with her when we visited. I imagine this was a godsend to her. We laughed and joked and talked about school and sports and what was going on in our lives at home. She kept the conversation very light. I believe she did so to keep her sanity, and to keep from breaking down in tears. When we prepared to leave, she welled up with emotion, and hugged me longer and more tightly than she ever had. "Things are going to be different when I get home, Babe," she said to me. "Better, much better." I looked at the tears running down her face. "Then why are you crying?" I asked, as I felt my own eyes water. "I just miss you Melin, I miss all of you guys," Mum said. "This place is going to make me better, but at the same time it's very difficult. I'm going to do it, though. I promise." She wiped her face. "Do me a huge favor, Sweetheart…pray for me. I really need it." My mother always had an intense faith in God, so I knew how important this request was to her. Squeezing her, I whispered, "I promise, Mum."

There is an expression I've heard, "Prayer is something we do in our time, the answers come in God's time." This was undoubtedly true in the case of my mother and her struggles. After a six month stretch of sobriety after rehab, Mum fell into relapse. It seemed as if nothing could keep her from continually falling back into her habit. My parents' marriage began to collapse. The arguments were constant. When they weren't fighting, they weren't talking. My father had recently purchased a property about two miles up the road from our house, which he was renovating to rent. Two weeks after school ended, my mother packed the car with games, food, sheets, and blankets and took my brothers and me on a "mini vacation" to this new house. We thought it was awesome; staying in a newly remodeled home, right across the street from our favorite hang out, closer to many of our friends. It was like a party. Again, because of our ages, not once did we even question this scenario. It didn't cross our minds that most married couples would not choose to live separately. One night, after staying up late playing board games with us, Mum sat me, Jimmy, and Matt down for a sobering conversation about her relationship with Dad. Once again, I was blindsided. She told us that she and my father were considering getting separated. "Divorced?" my brothers and I asked simultaneously. "No, not divorced. Just separated. Dad and I would still be married but

we'd just separate for a little while…to figure some things out."
"Does that mean you wouldn't live together anymore?" Jimmy
asked. "Yes, for a while anyway," she said as she kneeled in closer
to us. I couldn't believe what I was hearing. The thought of my
parents not living together changed my world. In my eyes, it
meant not only the separation of their marriage but of our family
as a whole. "Are you sure, Mum…isn't there some other way
to fix things?" I asked. My mother looked at me, knowing that
although this news was difficult for all of us, my kinship with
Dad may have made it especially hurtful for me. She took a deep
breath and carefully chose her words. "We're sure, Sweetie. Dad
and I have talked about this and right now this is the best thing
for us…and for you guys." Somehow I found it hard to believe
that we'd be better off in the proposed situation. "It doesn't mean
that we don't love each other anymore. We love each other very
much. And we love the three of you more than anything else
in the world, and that's the most important thing for you to
remember in all of this." I felt my face flushing with sadness, and
I tried my best to keep from crying. "This is none of your faults.
It's our decision. That being said, we want you all to be happy.
We think it would be best to have all of you live together with
one of us, either me or Dad, but we don't want to force you to
do something you don't want to do either. Of course you'd get to
see both of us all the time; it's just the living situation that needs
to be decided." I was unprepared for what she said next. "So we
thought it would be best for you to live with me, but if any of
you would prefer to live with Dad, then that would be fine too,"
she said. Although it wasn't a question, Mum was clearly looking
for a response from us. I instinctively looked to my brothers for
their reaction, even though I knew what their preferences would
be. Of the three of us, my little brother Matt had always been the
closest to my mother. He was her baby in every respect. Even at
his very young age, Matthew understood Mum on a very deep
level, as she did him. They were buddies for life and there was no

way he'd rather live with my father than with her. Jimmy was also extremely tight with Mum. He was a very unique and delicate soul as a little boy, and his individuality resulted in years of being picked on and bullied at school. My mother was very much his protector. His nature also caused him to be somewhat fearful of Dad and his fiery temper. For these reasons, I knew my older brother would also prefer to live with Mum. "I want to be with you," Matt said almost instantly. "Me too," Jimmy echoed. An awkward silence followed his comment, as I hesitated to answer. I'd been Daddy's little girl (or tomboy) since the day I was born, and I couldn't imagine not playing catch with him after dinner, or not watching the game with him at night. At the time, those were some of the most important things in my life. He was my hero. Not that I didn't idolize my mother as well; I loved her deeply. I simply felt a stronger bond, at that point in my life, with my father. I stared at the floor to avoid eye contact with either her or my siblings. "Melin?" Mum said. "What would you want to do?" Feeling immense pressure and panic, I responded impulsively, not thinking of how my answer would affect her feelings. "I think I might want to live with Dad," I muttered under my breath, my head still lowered. As soon as the words came out of my mouth I felt a sickness in the pit of my stomach at the thought of making my mother sad. I feared looking up at her; I thought for sure she'd be crying. To my relief, she was not. Instead, she calmly nodded at me with knowing eyes, as if anticipating my answer. "Melin!? No!" my brothers retorted. "That means we won't be together. You can't!" Mum immediately put and end to their comments. "Hey, guys…there will be none of that. If that's what would make her most happy then we'll respect her wishes. And that's that." I was thankful for her response, but still worried that I'd hurt her. I've often wondered how difficult it must have been for her to have responded in such a selfless manner, without judgment or questioning. Although she apparently managed to remove her ego from the situation, I know her feelings must have been deeply affected. She did so, however, because she was an incredible mother.

The topic was soon changed, as I believe Mum sensed how unsettled we'd become. I also believe she needed to escape discussion of this impending reality and the changes it would inevitably bring. Somehow, as only she could do, she had us in stitches by the end of the night. Mum always said laughter was the best medicine. I'd never fully understood this saying until that moment, and had never been so grateful for it either. Her laughter was a well needed bandage. As I closed my eyes in rest that evening, I heard my mother quietly cry herself to sleep.

CHAPTER 9

An Unexpected Sobriety

A FEW DAYS LATER, WE PACKED THE STATION WAGON AND HEADED DOWN the Cape for our annual summer trip. Having reluctantly absorbed the possibility that our parents might separate, my bothers and I were happy to get away for a couple weeks, and a vacation on Cape Cod with Mum would provide the perfect dose of amnesia. We were about half way through our holiday when my mother told us she had to go home for a day, and that our Aunt Mary was going to watch us in her absence. Because she mentioned it so nonchalantly, none of us really thought much of her announcement. When Jimmy asked why she had to leave, Mum simply responded that she had to take care of something at home, and that she'd be back by the end of the day. Aunt Mary was my mother's oldest sister and had been a nun for nearly forty years. She had no children of her own, so she loved spoiling her nieces and nephews with infinite varieties of junk food. Needless to say, we welcomed her with open arms.

As promised, Mum returned to the cottage later that night. We must have been a sight to see. Blissfully losing consciousness from food coma, my brothers and I lay like little beached whales on the living room floor, barely able to keep our eyes open to watch television. Falling in and out of sleep, I vaguely heard my mother and aunt whispering in the kitchen next door. I wasn't in any condition to register what was being said. When I woke the next morning, however, I recalled dreaming of Aunt Mary hugging Mum and holding her hand, and telling her that God would watch over her. Because I was used to having very vivid dreams, I didn't even question whether this consolation had actually taken place. I assumed the images of my aunt comforting my mother were probably in relation to my parents' potential upcoming marital changes. Subconsciously I may have been thinking about why my mother had to leave us that afternoon. She had gone home for the day, so maybe she and Dad had argued again. How I wish my little scenario had been the case. As we finished our vacation, I noticed a difference in this woman who typically reveled in her time on the Cape. Her laugh was gone. Something was off.

To my delight, there was no talk of Mum and Dad separating when we returned home. Everything seemed back to normal; we were all living together under one roof, and my parents seemed very tender toward one another. I happily avoided the dreaded topic. Maybe they made up? Maybe the "time apart" Mum had referred to had just passed? Maybe they changed their minds? Whatever the reason, I couldn't have been happier. The calm before the storm.

It's strange, of all the recollections in my life, both small and monumental, you'd think one of the memories I would remember most clearly is the exact moment when I learned my mother had breast cancer. Oddly enough, I can't. It was a process over several weeks; perhaps months. Mum left us down the Cape that afternoon because she had gone to have a lump in her breast examined. Her sister Kay had died from the disease nine years earlier at the age of forty, so Mum was understandably shaken by her unwanted discovery. Because her primary physician was on vacation through Labor Day, her appointment was with one of his colleagues, with whom she was unfamiliar. Whether he was simply trying to put her mind at ease or perhaps just rushing through his patients that day, he didn't seem to hold much stock in my mother's concerns, particularly regarding prior family history. The doctor vaguely concluded that the lump was most likely due to changes in my mother's menstrual cycle. Even though Mum questioned his pseudo diagnosis several times before leaving the office, and stressed the fact that her sister had died at such a young age from breast carcinoma, the physician still told her that it was (and I quote), "Nothing to worry about." No biopsies. No tests. Nothing. She was told to enjoy the rest of her vacation and to schedule an appointment with her regular doctor when he returned. So she did, reluctantly. I wasn't dreaming when I overheard Aunt Mary consoling Mum, when she told her that God would protect her and that everything would be fine. Neither had I imagined that things had noticeably changed between my parents; that they were expressing more love and concern for each other than they had in years. Unfortunately the catalyst for both of these situations was my mother's misdiagnosis. There was about a two month interval between her initial visit with the fill-in doctor and the first available appointment with her own physician. When Mum finally saw her primary doctor, he was shocked by the cavalier manner in which his counterpart had handled her condition, and immediately ordered the appropriate diagnostic tests. Despite his expeditious efforts, the damage had already been done. Quite literally. At a time when she thought life was bringing about difficult but manageable change, Mum was handed a brand new reality. One which would change her, and us, forever. It was unbearably sobering.

CHAPTER 10

The Power of Perception

Perhaps one of the reasons I can't accurately recall the exact moment when I discovered Mum had breast cancer is because she made a conscious effort not to use the term "cancer" when she spoke about her illness with me and my brothers. "Cancer," in itself, has to be one of the most feared terms in modern language. To children, it is not a disease state, or something that can be maintained or managed. Cancer is a reason someone dies. At least it was in 1990, when my mother was diagnosed. Mindful of this, Mum would instead refer simply to a "lump in her breast;" one for which there was no cause for us to panic. She also told us, with great enthusiasm, that she had a wonderful team of doctors who were going to help her get rid of it. A couple simple surgeries and some minor treatments were needed, which

Mum reassured us were no big deal. At fourteen, twelve, and ten years old, my brothers and I were fairly calm with this picture our mother painted, and came to very safe conclusions regarding her condition. Such is the power of perception. *Ok, so it's not cancer then, it's just a lump. How hard can it be to remove a lump? Mum's just sick again.* So although not completely ignorant to the situation, we were blissfully unaware of its complexity. In a way I'm thankful for this unknowingness, as it protected us tremendously. Our unfamiliarity with the real possibilities and consequences related to our mother's circumstance kept us from a heightened level of worry and anguish; one far more absolute. I can legitimately say that I didn't even realize my mother had actual "breast cancer" until a few months later, when I overheard two of my teachers discussing it in the break room at school. Mum had been sick and in the hospital several times throughout our lives, so it wasn't a stretch for us to believe that this was just another bout with illness, or for us to group this together with conditions such as high blood pressure or colitis.

On the other hand, I often wish I had been older and more educated on the situation when it happened, so I could have discussed the options with my mother, woman to woman. Advancements in the field of breast cancer, in terms of research, prevention, education, diagnostics, and treatment, have radically progressed since 1990, when my mother was diagnosed. Possibilities such as genetic testing did not exist, and procedures such as mastectomies were viewed as last resort options. Most women avoided such surgeries out of vanity, as "breast reconstruction" was not readily available at the time. Lumpectomies, chemotherapy, and radiation were the standard of care. Public perception of the condition has changed as well. The disease used to carry a certain stigma which, thanks to public figures like Melissa Etheridge and Sheryl Crow, has been shed and transformed in recent years. For example, very rarely in the 1980's or 1990's would a woman with breast cancer be seen in public with a bald head. Equally as unlikely would be a patient wearing a stylish bandana instead of a wig, or rallying with her friends to participate in a three-day walk to find a cure. That's because these things didn't exist twenty years ago! Women have been empowered by these medical and social advances. I just wish the reality and understanding of this disease was then what it is now. Things may have been very different.

CHAPTER 11

Attitude

Everything happens for a reason. We've all heard this truism, right? Had it not been for my mother, I probably never would have found much credibility in it. There are people who cite this expression as a convenient cliché when they hear about something awful that happened to someone else. They typically drop this phrase not because they believe in it, but rather because they can't bear to face the fact that bad things sometimes happen to good people, and this is their method of rationalization. They say it more for their own selfish reassurance than for anything else. Or they might just be attempting to sound profound. On the other hand, there are individuals who truly see an interconnectedness within life. They genuinely believe that there is a master plan; that there are no coincidences; nothing, whether good *or* bad, occurs by accident. Ironically, these people are typically those who have experienced tragedy firsthand, who arguably have the most reason to complain or be angry with the world. Most likely, they were not born with such convictions, but instead developed them over years of realizing the interwoven nature of events, and finding purpose within them.

After the initial shock of her diagnosis, Mum's attitude toward her sickness was remarkably positive. She approached the disease with vigor, never once pitying herself. "What good is complaining going to do? Why bitch?" she would say. "You can either spend your time feeling sorry for yourself or you can do something about it. You can either laugh or cry about it. This thing is either gonna kick my ass or I'm gonna kick its ass. I'm planning on the latter. Either way, I'd rather be laughing." My mother walked the walk, too. She never grumbled about her condition. Instead she pointed out "blessings" that became of the situation. Mum and Dad reunited in a way I thought I'd never see. Their reconciliation was not spawned by guilt or obligation, but rather by much needed perspective. My parents had been chipping away at one another for the past few years, for reasons both trivial and significant. Each had nearly lost sight of the other, and the reasons for which they fell in love. My mother's cancer, quite frankly, scared the hell out of them, as most potentially life-threatening illnesses will do. Almost instantly, they put aside their differences and reprioritized their relationship. In doing so they were reborn with one another, and formed an unbreakable bond. "God has a funny way of making things happen, Melin," she said to me. "Have you ever noticed that you can't see the stars until night falls? Darkness is what makes stars visible."

Las Vegas was one of my parents' favorite vacation spots. They developed their love of Sin City in the early 1970's, when my mother worked for the airlines. Her job enabled them to travel frequently, and Vegas was arguably the most exciting place to be at the time. After my brothers and I were born, their trips to

"The Strip" were gradually replaced by family holidays to Disney World. About halfway through her first round of chemotherapy, Mum decided she wanted to get away for a few days. The treatment was taking its toll on her. The drugs that are available today, which assist in dulling the side effects of this therapy, were not available when my mother was battling cancer. As a result, she suffered from violent nausea and fatigue. Despite her condition, she insisted that she and Dad take a four day weekend to their old stomping grounds. Her attitude was that if she was going to be sick anyway, that she may as well be sick in a place where she'd be having fun. "I'll be fine Jim," she said. "I really just need to forget about this for a few days." That's all Dad needed to hear. He'd been seeing her go through hell, and wanted to provide relief in any way he could.

My brothers and I stayed with my aunt and uncle while my parents journeyed back to a place which held very happy memories for them. I think they needed to remember that joy and innocence, if only for a short while. Sometimes it takes revisiting an old friend or an old place to provide reminders of the things that were once good; and offer hope of that which can be even better. Naturally my father was concerned for my mother, and told her on their way there to take it easy and relax. "If I wanted to relax Monk, I'd have had you take me to the Caribbean. I'm here to have fun! And I don't want you worrying about me the whole time, either. The best thing you can do for me is just have a blast... *with* me." So even though he knew he would be concerned about her the entire time, my dad made a conscious effort to respect her wishes. And he did. When they arrived in Vegas, Mum and Dad were like kids in a candy store. Adrenaline kicked in, and Mum had newfound energy. She and my father partied as they had years before. It was as if they were newlyweds again. For a moment, they were completely carefree; without responsibilities or harsh realities. On their second night of vacation, however, reality came calling. My parents were in their hotel room getting ready to go downstairs to gamble for the night. As Dad came out of the shower, he saw Mum combing her hair in front of the mirror. "Oh no," he heard her say. Walking toward her, my father saw the physical evidence of her dismay. Clumps of hair had been combed out in her brush. She stopped for a minute and looked at my Dad. Gazing back toward her reflection, she delicately ran her hand over her scalp. Even more hair. There was silence. No words needed to be spoken between my parents, as they were both thinking the same thing. *It's starting.* After a brief moment of absorption, Mum reacted in a way only she could. "We knew this was coming, right?" she said to Dad. "I just need a few minutes by myself, Monk...if you don't mind." My father resisted at first. "Marian, I'm not going anywhere. I really should be with you right now." "I appreciate that Sweetie, but its fine...I just need a few moments by myself," she replied. "Tell you what, go downstairs, find a good spot at the table, and I'll meet you down there in fifteen minutes." He refused. "No way, I am *not* leaving you right now." "Please," she said. "I'm asking you. It will be ok. I will be down in two seconds...I promise." He agreed reluctantly, only because he wanted to honor her request.

Although his mind couldn't have been further from gambling, my father went to the casino and pulled up a seat at the craps table as Mum had suggested. Checking his watch about every thirty seconds, he waited. As ten minutes approached, he started to push his chair away from the table. Standing up to leave, he looked up and saw my mother walking towards him. Smirking bashfully, she lifted her hands up toward her head as if to ask, "*What do you think?*" In anticipation of her hair falling out, Mum had purchased a wig the week before the trip, and brought it with her just in case. Not missing a beat, she'd combed out the rest of her hair and donned her new locks. When Mum reached the table, she leaned over and kissed my father. "So are we winning?" she said, as she rubbed his back. Dad just stared. He was overwhelmed by her. Her resilience. Her strength. Her courage. He'd never loved her as much as he did in that moment. She had redefined beauty.

My aunt brought us to the airport to pick up my parents upon their return. As soon as I saw my mother, I noticed something different about her, though I couldn't pinpoint it. She looked excited but slightly nervous as she approached us. I'm sure she sensed our curiosity. Neither my brothers nor I asked about her new hairdo. In retrospect, I believe we may have intentionally avoided doing so. Several weeks passed before we were actually made aware that Mum was wearing a wig. Always with her kids in mind, my mother went out of her way several times throughout her illness in order to keep our lives as normal as possible. This included her avoidance of the term "cancer" in the early stages of her battle, not mentioning her wig until we asked, and specifically never letting us see her bald head. Mum was very conscious of the fact that certain things would make her disease more tangible to us, so she went to great lengths to keep specific details hidden in an attempt to protect us. I would not learn of or fully appreciate her acts of selflessness until years later. As much as I admired Mum for her verbal and expressive abilities, I've come to realize many of the things that made her an amazing mother were done in silence.

CHAPTER 12

Faith Lost

AUGUST 19, 1991. MUM, MY BROTHERS, AND I WERE ENJOYING OUR LAST days of vacation on the Cape. Hurricane Bob made landfall, and my mother used the Category Three storm as an excuse to have a "hurricane party." We all went outside to take pictures and were nearly blown away down the street. Of course this was hysterical to us. We were laughing so hard we could barely find the strength to grab on to something and get back inside the house. Mum somehow managed to capture the whole thing on film. Because we had no electricity, she ventured to make pasta in a pan over a charcoal grill. To say it was one of the top five worst meals ever would be kind. Jimmy, Matt, and I tried to hide our disgust at first, forcing the mushy spaghetti into our mouths. We couldn't heat the sauce so we used ketchup. It was just gross, but none of us wanted to hurt Mum's feelings. After a couple bites, she looked up to gage our reaction. We chewed in repulsed silence. Quite aware of our revulsion, she asked out of her own amusement, "How is it guys... not bad, huh?" The three of us looked at each other and knew we had to lie. She'd made such a valiant effort. "It's great Mum," we answered in staggered unison. I could practically feel my nose growing as I uttered my response. My mother took the opportunity to have some fun with us. "I've never thought of making pasta this way, but it's just so good...and with ketchup....who would have thought! I think I'll make it this way from now on!" My brothers and I almost choked on our food. What had we done!? It must have looked like we'd seen a ghost. Mum wasn't the greatest cook to begin with, but she had really outdone herself this time. The texture of the meal alone made me nauseous. I could barely look at her, as I was sure she'd be able to see my queasiness. Without warning, my mother burst into laughter. It took us a second to realize she'd been putting us on; that she was as sickened by her own cooking as we were. "You guys are priceless...and horrible liars, but I love you for it." When she was done cracking herself up, she dumped the rest of the gooey mess into the trash. With not many options left, Mum went into the kitchen and grabbed a couple bags of Doritos and a box of Little Debbie cakes. "Desperate times..." she said, smiling at us. Jimmy, Matt and I were in heaven. For the rest of the night, we sat around the fire eating junk food and making fun of our mother's meal. It was blissful.

August 23, 1991. The hurricane had passed and the power had come back on, and we'd just finished packing the cooler for a day at the beach. Just as we were leaving the cottage, the phone rang. Turning around to answer it, Mum told us to wait in the car and that she'd be right out. Jimmy, Matt and I waited impatiently for what seemed like an eternity, but in actuality was about five minutes. Eventually we headed back inside, wondering what was taking our mother so long. She was hanging up just as we walked in the door. "Ok, Mary...I'm on my way. I'll be there as soon as

I can." Her voice cracked with emotion, and she had panic in her eyes. "What's wrong, Mum?" Matt asked. "Pack your stuff, guys. We're going home. Now." Like most kids would react, we thought nothing of what our mother's conversation had entailed, but instead only of the fact that, for some reason, our vacation was being cut short. "What! Why?" we asked in whining voices. She walked away from us and into her bedroom, opened her closet, took out her suitcase, and immediately started packing her clothes. Her sense of urgency was unsettling. I stood timidly in the doorway of her room as I watched her frantically gather her belongings. "What's wrong Mum? What is it?" I asked. I knew something bad had happened, but I'd never seen her react in such a way, even to her own illness. "Pa's in the hospital. He's had a stroke." My Pa (my mother's father) was one of my favorite people in the world. To my mum, he was the world. Although I didn't fully understand what a stroke was at the time, I knew enough to know that one could be deadly. "Is it bad?" I said, starting to panic myself. Mum's eyes started to fill with tears. "I don't know, Pumpkin, I just want to get home so I can be with him." Jim and Matt overheard our conversation. With no further explanation necessary, we quickly collected our things.

When we arrived home, my mother made sure my brothers and I had enough food to make a simple dinner for ourselves, then promptly headed into Boston with my father. Dad called once in the early evening to make sure we were alright. When I asked him how Pa was doing, my father answered vaguely. "Not so great, Sweetie." While this response was certainly not what I wanted to hear, I could not have imagined the news we'd receive upon my parents' return late that night. My grandfather had passed away. He'd suffered a massive stroke caused by a subarachnoid hemorrhage. He was eighty-six years old.

When my mother and father walked through the door, they were silent. Mum looked weak with grief, her eyes almost lifeless. Dad was gently supporting her with his arms, as if she might faint if he let go. She started to bawl uncontrollably as soon as she saw us. She was inconsolable. I'd never seen anyone weep so hard or so deeply. She was heartbroken. Eventually my father took my mother upstairs and did all he could to comfort her. When he came downstairs, he started to explain to us what had happened. Pa had never regained consciousness, so although the entire family was with him when he passed, Mum never had a final chance to speak with him or say goodbye. "That's all she kept saying to me in the car on the way home," Dad said. "She just kept saying, 'I never got a chance to say goodbye to him, Jim. I just wish I could have told him I loved him one last time.'" Suddenly our discussion was interrupted by the sound of glass smashing. We heard our mother, from the top of the stairs, screaming at the top of her lungs. "I hate you!!! I hate you!!! How could you do this to me? I frigging hate you!!!" We all ran into the foyer, to see what had happened and at whom she was yelling. My first reaction was to look up toward Mum. She was slumped over the banister, sobbing intensely. For a second I was confused. I initially thought she may have been shouting at my late grandfather for dying. Then my gaze descended from my mother to the floor below her. There, lying in shattered pieces, was a picture of Jesus Christ. It had been a staple on Mum's nightstand for as long as I could remember. I went numb for a moment. I didn't know what to think. My mother was one of the most religious people I'd ever known, so hearing her curse the very thing she believed in most was devastating; frightening even. As scared as I was, I couldn't bear to see her in such pain. Instinctively, I climbed the stairs and wrapped my arms around her. My dad and brothers followed; hugging her, kissing her, and rubbing her back. Although I was deeply saddened by Pa's death, all I could think of in that moment was my mum. Had she lost her faith? For as much doubt raced through my mind, one thing was for certain. As agonizing as that moment was, I'd never felt so close to my family.

CHAPTER 13

A Rapid Decline

My grandfather's death catalyzed a cascade of sorrow for my mother. She'd lost one of her best friends in life, her faith was in question, and her medical condition was worsening. After nearly two years of successful lumpectomies, chemotherapy, and radiation treatments, her cancer seemed to be heading toward remission. Soon after her tragic loss, however, we learned that her illness was recurrent. Mum had a catheter placed permanently in her chest in order to administer controlled release chemotherapy. As a result, she was sick and physically exhausted a large majority of the time, although she tried desperately to conceal it. Years later, I learned that Mum's oncologist told my father that her case was "the single worst case of breast cancer" he'd ever seen.

To make matters worse, our family, as close as we'd been while consoling our mother through Pa's death, had changed dramatically. My brother Jimmy was rebelling to years of frustration from being picked on and abused by bullying classmates. Like most teenagers who harbor such forced disdain, he inadvertently released his rage on those he cared about most, his family. My brother's anger and Dad's temper were a disastrous combination. They had horrific fights, both verbal and physical. It made for a constantly argumentative and hostile environment. My mother hired a therapist to come to the house once a week. Her visits were some of the most awkward experiences of my life. Despite her best efforts, her methods were very generic, so needless to say her textbook solutions as to how we could "reconnect" as a family failed. We tried other options. Group counseling. Therapy. Unfortunately nothing seemed to work. The stress in our household was at an all time high. Finally, after nearly a year of unbearable confrontation, my parents opted for the very last resort of temporarily placing my older brother in a foster home. It was a gut-wrenching decision, but they felt that it was the right one considering my mother's declining health. Mum felt powerless, as if she'd lost all control in her life. Control of her health. Control of her family. Control of her fate. If ever she was tested, it was then. Finding herself in the greatest state of helplessness she'd ever known, she did the only thing she believed could truly save her at that point. She turned back to her faith.

CHAPTER 14

Faith Reborn

It is a rare but beautiful thing to see someone you love experience a spiritual awakening. Although it didn't take place overnight, my mother rekindled her relationship with God, and in doing so created a renewed understanding of faith. Her beliefs were now far more spiritual than religious. She focused on the fundamental teachings of Jesus rather than the rules and formalities imposed by the institution of the church. It was a subtle but notable difference. My mother was never a slave to traditions, and this included those associated with Catholicism. She was a believer and practiced certain customs as a result of her upbringing, but Mum was equally comfortable speaking with God in the comfort of her own home or while taking a walk on the beach as she was at Mass. She used to tell me that it didn't matter where

I was or whom I was with; that I was always with God and He was always with me, and therefore there were no restrictions as to when or where I could pray. She also stressed that the core of any religion is faith and spirituality, not customs or protocol. This was a much welcomed balance to some of the opposing views I'd heard during my years of parochial schooling. She built a mini shrine which included my grandfather's Mass card, a newly framed picture of Jesus Christ, her rosary beads, and holy water from Knock, Ireland. This sanctuary was portable, and she took it down the Cape with us that summer on vacation. Many times, unbeknownst to her, I would watch and listen to her pray. It was never the same twice. Sometimes she would have full blown conversations, other times she would whisper, and then there were times when she would remain in complete silence for hours at a time. Mum seemed to be at a higher level of peace and comfort than I had ever seen her before, even prior to her cancer. I never asked my mother what prompted her enlivening, but I suspect the reality of her condition forced her to grasp her own mortality, and therefore caused her to seek her true convictions regarding life after death. Whether or not this was the catalyst, she seemed to have found genuine serenity, and by this I was inspired. Her example during this time is very much the basis of my own faith.

In her rejuvenation, Mum found even more strength and vivacity than she'd previously possessed. There is one particular event, which until now has been a private memory between me and my mother, which epitomizes her courage and passion for life. Our cousins from Ireland were in Boston visiting for two weeks. Mum had been very ill, but had done her best to camouflage her failing health to her relatives. To celebrate our guests' final night in town, the entire extended family planned on attending an event at one of the most well-known Irish dance halls in the city. Nothing could have been a better and more needed night out for my mother. She loved Irish music and dance more than anyone. She'd been raised on it. It was as much a part of her as her humor and intelligence, and she passed her passion for it not only to her children, but to her Italian husband as well. We were all looking forward to this night.

As I was getting dressed for the evening, Mum called for me from the bathroom. "Melin, can you come here for a minute?" I walked out of my room and toward the bathroom, two doors down. When I opened the door, I immediately saw crimson dripping down the counter onto the floor. My first thought was that my mother had been painting her nails and perhaps spilled some of the polish. As I walked further into the bathroom, however, the bathtub in which my mother was sitting came into sight. She looked up at me with calmness in her eyes, as if to avert the panic which she knew would overcome me. There was blood everywhere. *Everywhere.* On her hands. On the floor. In the tub. On the doorknob of the linen closet. Her legs were wrapped in towels that had once been white, but were now soaked deep red. Wondering what had happened, I frantically began to ask, "Mum, what…" Before I could even complete my question, she intervened. In a completely casual voice, she said, "It looks a lot worse than it really is, Babe. Can you come over here for a second? I need you to do something for me. Close the door first." Although utterly confused, I was eased by her peaceful tone. "Do me a favor and grab the big beach towels at the top of the closet." Stretching my body to reach the shelf they were on, I yanked down the towels to which she was referring. I quickly brought them to the tub and knelt down next to her. Instinctively, I began to remove the blood drenched cloths that were covering her legs to replace them with these new ones. "No, Sweetie," she said, as she took the linens from me. Mum rolled the towels into balls and placed one on her thighs and the other on her shins. "I need you to sit on me, on my legs…to help stop the bleeding." Still not knowing what had caused the bloodshed, I did as my mother requested. As I climbed into the bathtub with her, she patted her quads, motioning me to sit just above her knees. I lowered myself delicately, as I did not want to hurt her. "I need all of you, skinny-minny," she said, pulling my entire weight down onto her limbs. "Now press down on my shins with your hands, Melin." As I pushed down, I could actually feel how saturated the towels she'd been using had become. I removed them, reached out of the tub, and grabbed two clean ones which I wrapped tightly around her calves. I pressed down on them with all my strength, while the rest of my body was putting pressure on her upper legs. Suddenly I felt my mother's hand on my back. "That a girl. Thanks, Pumpkin," she sighed, as she rubbed my head. I turned to her. "What happened, Mum?" "I did something I wasn't supposed to do," she started. "I'm on blood thinners, babe. I have to take them as part of my therapy. One of the risks in taking them is that they can cause me to bleed more easily. So my doctor told me not to shave." I looked to the edge of the tub and saw the razor. "I started bleeding with the first stroke, but I just figured it would stop if I put a little pressure on it. I just wanted to get both legs done so I could wear a skirt tonight. I know it sounds stupid but I just wanted to dress up a little, you know? Just for tonight...I just wanted to shave my legs, put a skirt on, dress up and feel pretty again. Just for a night. I always wear a dress or a skirt when I go dancing." Even though I was only fourteen years old, and still a tomboy who loathed the thought of wearing a skirt, I understood what my mother was saying. She wanted to feel normal again, and beautiful again. If only just for a night.

For the first time, I felt a connection with her which transcended the mother-daughter relationship I'd always known. I saw her as more than my mother. I saw her as a woman. And although our tastes and distastes for fashion differed, the inherent desire to feel beautiful was the same. The cancer had taken its toll on her. She'd lost her hair on two separate occasions, she'd had multiple lumpectomies; her once vibrant and firm frame had become fragile and weakened. For as crazy and wild and mischievous as she was, Mum was always the epitome of femininity to me. She was a lady. Her charm was not in ever-proper etiquette or fine-tuned conversations. Her authenticity is what drew people to her; her humor, her sincerity and kindness, her passion for life. It was the way she made everyone around her feel completely comfortable. That's why people loved her. That's what made her a true lady. I looked directly at her. "That doesn't sound stupid at all, Mum. Not at all." Although I can't remember the exact content of the discussion we entered into after that, I do remember my mother making me laugh so hard that, had there been more room in the bathtub, I would have fallen off her legs. She was cracking jokes at her own expense, as she always did. Mum always said that the ability to laugh at oneself was one of the greatest measures of self-confidence. It also made it permissible to laugh at others, which was one of her favorite pastimes. "As long as no one's feelings get hurt, it's ok" she'd say. To say the least, my mother had no lack of laughter in her life.

Eventually, we managed to get Mum's bleeding under control. As planned, she donned a gorgeous outfit which showed off her marvelous legs. She looked stunning. That night was one of the greatest of my life. Mostly, I think it was seeing my mother in old but rare form. Full of energy. Singing at the top of her lungs. Laughing so hard she lost her breath. Dancing like she owned the floor. She was in her element, and I was in awe of her. I remember watching her light up the room that night, and thinking that she was the bravest person I'd ever known, or ever would know for that matter. No one else had any clue what she had gone through just hours earlier. Mum would never mention it either, as she didn't want anyone to feel sorry for her, or be worried about her. She simply wanted to live that evening to its fullest. And she did…like there was no tomorrow.

And I had a new definition of hero.

CHAPTER 15

Transition

IN EARLY DECEMBER 1992 MY PARENTS HEADED TO LAS VEGAS TO celebrate my Dad's forty-fourth birthday in style, complete with tickets to see Frank Sinatra, who shared a birthday with my father and happened to be performing in Sin City to commemorate his eightieth year. My mother was very ill at the time, and her doctors actually advised her against traveling in such a delicate state. Mum, as expected, was defiant. Her attitude again was that if she was sick anyway, that she may as well be so in a place where she was having fun instead of sitting at home feeling badly for herself. More than that, and I've come to realize this in recent years, I think she knew exactly how serious her condition had become, and wanted to make the most of her time.

I was only a few months into my freshman year of high school and was staying with my Aunt Eileen while my parents were out of town. Her daughter (my cousin) Nikki was a year ahead of me in grade, but light years beyond me in terms of adjustment to the social nuances that came along with entering high school. I absolutely *hated* my first few months at Cardinal Spellman High. As a tomboy, I felt very awkward in my new surroundings. The girls all seemed much older, prettier, and more physically developed than I. While this alone was enough to make me feel uncomfortable, my personal insecurity stemmed from the cruelty of others. Before then, I'd never been aware of anything about myself that would be cause for concern or embarrassment. It only took a couple of months of high school and a few scarring comments on my hair, my acne, my flat chest, and my boyishness to make me very self-conscious.

This was a very difficult transition from the loving, unpretentious environment in which Mum and Dad had raised me. I'd always felt entirely secure in my own skin, as my parents had continually supported my individuality throughout my life. They knew who I was and they let me be so. There was never any pressure to become more feminine or attempt more stereotypically female activities. Mum always said that if I ever were to have interest in such things that it would come in my own time, not anyone else's. And as prophesized, my initial curiosity in "girly" things began shortly before entering Spellman. Although I realize she was probably thrilled that I was finally showing attentiveness in areas in which she and I could bond, my mother was also careful to not place a huge emphasis on physicality. Mum would let me borrow her clothes (she and I were about the same height at the time) and her jewelry. She also gave me a very basic introduction to makeup, stressing the importance of subtlety. "The way you'll know you're wearing it correctly is if no one can tell you have it on," she'd say. "A little bit to highlight your features, Melin, but don't ever cover up what God painted. Natural is beautiful." Because my mother went at my pace, I really enjoyed this new facet of my relationship with her. And for that very reason, combined with my harsh introduction to life as a high schooler, I needed her back home.

Besides the kinship I had formed with my new and only friend Trevor, who remains dear to me to this day, I had nothing to look forward to when I went to school. I was counting down the days until my parents' return. On the morning they were to head home, I woke up with a bounce in my step. I just couldn't wait to see them. Aunt Eileen was supposed to drive me back to our house in Stoughton after school, as Mum and Dad were scheduled to have arrived by then. Instead, she drove me back to her house in Brockton. "There's been a little change of plans, Hon," she said. I thought perhaps my parents were coming to pick me up at her place, and that's why we had returned there. "Your mum and dad are back, but they needed to go straight to the hospital." She was doing her best to sound calm. "Your mother started to get sick at the end of the trip, so they thought it would be best to go right to the hospital instead of going home first." Although I was relatively composed, most in thanks to my aunt's deliberate effort to keep me so, I was inwardly unnerved. "Is she ok?" I asked, knowing that although she was making a conscious attempt to act casually, Eileen would never mislead me if I questioned her directly. She looked me straight in the eye, sensing my awareness. "I don't know…I hope so, Honey. That's why they went directly to the hospital. They didn't want to take any chances." *Any chances of what?* I thought to myself, but intentionally neglected to ask out loud. The date was December 13th.

CHAPTER 16

"Mummy's Really Sick This Time"

Mum had spent so much time in hospitals throughout her life, that her admittance on this occasion was not enough alone to cause inordinate concern. What alarmed me was the apparent urgency of the situation; the fact that my parents didn't even stop at home before going to the hospital. This is what worried me most. Although I did my best to rationalize, a dreaded but apparent reality kept entering in my mind. *It must be bad.* I needed to see her; to prove myself wrong.

New England Baptist Hospital in Boston, where Mum received all of her breast cancer treatment, was regarded as one of the leading hospitals in the area for oncology. This would be my first time visiting my mother within these walls. She'd been admitted the night before and, at her request, spent the evening alone with my father. The next day Dad picked up my brother Jimmy from St. Vincent's in Fall River, where he'd been staying for the past couple of months, and we all went in to see Mum together. We hadn't gathered in one place as a whole family in a long time, and although the circumstances weren't the best, I think we were all grateful. Within minutes of seeing my mother, I knew this wasn't like any of her other stints at the hospital. Mum was heavily medicated and seemed completely out of it. Her speech was slurred and her eyes were unfocused. She was pale and looked more physically frail than I had ever seen her. I specifically recall her applying an ointment to her lips, which had dried out and cracked as a result of one of the meds she'd been taking. It seemed so painful. Even more heartbreaking was the fact that she seemed somewhat aware of her incoherence, and was trying desperately to hold normal conversations with us. Although we realized this was an entirely different type of inebriation, her incognizance was eerily similar to the drunken states in which we'd seen her so many times during her alcoholism. In a strange way, I wish she had been drunk. At that moment, it seemed like a much better option than what that damn cancer and its treatment was doing to her.

Christmas Eve, 1992. After about ten days in the hospital, my mother was scheduled to come home just in time for the holiday. We couldn't have been more thrilled. Dad was bringing her home that night, so Matt and I did our part getting the house cleaned and ready for her. We'd never been more motivated to do housework. Mum had only been in the hospital for a week and a half, but her absence, combined with my father's constant running back and forth to be with her, resulted in a very messy household being run by two kids. We'd unintentionally trashed our normally immaculate home, and for the first time we became aware of how hard Mum worked to keep things so beautiful. Within a matter of hours, the house was as good as new; vacuumed, dusted and shined. After cleaning, my brother and I poured some eggnog, put on the holiday music and began to decorate the Christmas tree. We were so excited for Mum to come home. This was always the happiest time of the year in our house. Our tradition was to exchange family gifts on the night before Christmas, as December twenty-fifth was dedicated solely for Santa's presents. Even though we were getting older, this custom never lost its magic. I couldn't wait to give Mum her gifts that night.

As the evening went on, my brother and I started to check the clock with growing anxiety. My father told us he and my mother would be home around six o'clock. Now nearly eight-thirty, Matt and I started to worry. I turned on the television as a distraction. As always, TBS was running "A Christmas Story" on a loop. Eternally captivated by this holiday classic, my brother and I sat down to watch. Within minutes, we heard the garage door opening. Matt and I flew up off of the living room floor and ran into the kitchen, our hearts pounding with excitement. When Dad walked in by himself, our exuberance quickly turned into confusion. "Where's Mum?" Matt immediately asked. My father paused for a brief moment, as if trying to think of something clever to say. He must have quickly realized that nothing of the sort could befit the situation. "Uh....she um...," he started to say. Our eyes met for a fleeting instant. He was clearly nervous and could not hold his gaze at me. "She can't come home tonight, Bud," he said to my brother. Both of our hearts sank. Before either of us could ask why, my Dad started leading us into the living room. "Let's sit down for a minute," he said gently, as he placed his hands on our shoulders. "The house looks great. Nice job, guys. Your mother would be very proud of you." Somehow his comments on our cleaning seemed like an attempt at small talk. My father didn't make small talk. Something was wrong.

As Matt and I sat down on the couch, Dad grabbed the remote control and shut off the TV. He clearly didn't want us distracted from what he was about to say. As he took his seat next to me, I could physically sense his tension. My father was the most emotional man I knew, and always wore his heart on his sleeve. It was one of the things I loved most about him. For better or for worse, I never had to guess how he was feeling. Unfortunately this time, it seemed very much like it was for the worse. There is a certain preparatory routine my dad goes through when he talks about something serious. He has a particular tone in his voice, one more delicate than that in which he normally speaks. Also, he always looks us directly in the eyes when speaking to us about important matters. In that instance, the lack of eye contact is what disturbed me most. From the time he came through the door, he avoided our eyes. Typically never at a loss for words, my father also struggled to speak. He would start then stop, rub his face with both hands and sigh, begin to speak then stop again. He was fidgeting and started to break out in a mild sweat. I'd never seen him like this. He could not find the words. Finally, he gathered himself. "Mummy's not coming home tonight because she's really sick this time...*really* sick." As I felt the blood rush to my face, Matt interjected. "How sick?" he asked. My father looked up at me for the first time. He was tightlipped and had tears in his eyes. Once again, he couldn't speak, and lowered his head toward the ground. The seconds that passed as I waited for his answer were the longest of my life. I simply didn't want him to respond. *Please tell us that they just want to keep her in the hospital to try a new medication*, I thought. *Or that she just needs more chemo or radiation...or that they're just sending her to a different hospital.* As much as I yearned to hear these explanations, I knew they weren't coming. A single tear streamed down Dad's face. Although I knew his prospective reply could change our world forever, I felt compelled to help him get it out. He was the strongest man I knew, yet seeing him cry and unable to speak forced me to ask the question I'd never seriously contemplated until that moment. "Is she dying?" I felt hollow as the words left my mouth. As I prepared for his answer, my mind went blank. The entire scenario was surreal. Then the silence was broken. My father looked directly into my eyes. In his tears, I saw his answer. "Yes," he said, as his voice broke with heartache. I felt a dull pain run through my entire body, and remember thinking that my heart, literally, must have been breaking. The numbness sent a tremor of emotion through my system, and I began to weep. Dad grabbed me and my brother and hugged us tightly. His own tears were now gone, as he was now focused on comforting his children. Barely able to think, only one question came to my mind. "How long does she have?" I asked my father, my face wet and pressed against his. "They said about three weeks," he whispered, rubbing the back of my head. With these words, terminality set in. Until that moment, I never believed that my mother would die from cancer. She had been "living with it," "fighting it," and "beating it" for nearly three years. How did it ever get to this point? The remainder of the evening was a blur to me. Though I was listening, I had difficulty fully comprehending the details of Mum's worsened diagnosis. I was deafened with grief, and had heard all I needed to hear.

Although I would not realize it until years later, perhaps due to my own dazedness when the conversation occurred, my younger brother did not register this news the same way I did. He was sitting right next to me, so he definitely heard it. Furthermore, Dad did not mince words, or give us an "everyone dies eventually" speech. So how was it then, that Matt didn't fully comprehend what our father had said? Whether it was a deliberate effort on his part, or if he just mentally shut down in anticipation of my father's disclosure, my little brother did not understand completely that my mother was going to die. To this day, I don't know whether to consider this a blessing or a curse. All I know was that Christmas Eve, 1992 was the worst night of my life.

CHAPTER 17

Christmas Morning, 1992

Like most children who celebrate Christmas, I arose unusually early on the morning of December twenty-fifth, perhaps unconsciously hardwired with the excitement typically associated with that day. Unlike past holidays however, when my brothers would bust into my room and pull me out of bed so we could run downstairs and open our gifts, I awoke in complete silence. I woke up facing the window as I usually did, having habitually slept on my left side. As I came to consciousness, I felt an immediate warmth on my face. The sun was shining directly into my room. My eyes adjusted to a brilliantly blue and cloudless sky. Lying there, I felt completely at peace. It wasn't often that I had the opportunity to experience such serenity in the morning. The dreaded alarm clock was not ringing, and my father was not brutishly banging down my door to tell me that I had to get up to get ready for school. Then it dawned on me. *It's Christmas.* Second only to my birthday, Christmas Day was undoubtedly my favorite occasion of the year. As quickly as my excitement started to build, however, it disappeared with uncertainty. Confused for a moment, I started to remember the events of the previous night. *Mummy's not coming home.* For a brief moment, I thought those words may have come to me in a dream. I rolled out of bed and walked over to the mirror. Unfortunately, my reflection brought me to my senses. My eyes were bloodshot with exhaustion; my face washed clean with tears. Suddenly I recalled crying myself to sleep. It hadn't been a dream. It was in fact a nightmare.

The smell of Christmas consumed me as I walked downstairs, thanks in part to the overwhelming aroma of pine from our tree. Dad, having been absorbed with shuttling back and forth to the hospital, had somehow managed to find time to pick it up for us on the previous afternoon. As I turned into the parlor, I was overtaken with sadness. I saw everything which symbolized what I had always associated with the holiday: the tree, the presents, the fire burning in the fireplace, the snow on the back deck. On this morning, however, Christmas was not there. Mum wasn't sitting on the couch in her oversized, furry pink bathrobe sipping on her third cup of tea, reveling in our happiness as we opened our gifts. Dad wasn't videotaping our faces as we laughed our way through the morning. The holiday music that had been the soundtrack to so many of our Christmas sunrises was not playing. On this beautiful and normally joyous occasion, I stood alone and empty. It started to hit me. My life, as I knew it, was coming to an end. Mum was dying. *She'll never be in this house again. She'll never be here for another Christmas.* Then I started to think further into the future. *She won't see me graduate high school or college. She won't see me fall in love or get married or have babies.* Everything I had ever imagined in life involved her. Now for the first time, I started to prepare myself for the grim reality of facing life without this wonderful woman who had become my best friend.

Thankfully, my solitude was broken by my father, who'd been sitting in the kitchen and heard me come downstairs. "Merry Christmas, Pumpkin," he said, as he wrapped his arms around me and kissed me on the cheek. The words were so familiar but the feeling was so different. "Merry Christmas, Dad." I embraced him more tightly than usual, and held onto him with every ounce of love I possessed. It struck me that I would inevitably have to endure the same daunting reality of losing him one day. The thought was too much for me to bear. When we finally came apart, we stood in silence for several seconds. No words were needed. Each of us knew what the other was thinking, and was grateful for the other's unspoken understanding. Matt came down a few moments later. His unaffectedness, although concerning, provided well needed normalcy. "Should we open gifts?" he asked. It dawned on all of us that we didn't really know what to do. Mum was in the hospital. Jimmy was in the boys' residential home. "Why don't we pack them up and take them to the hospital so we can open them with Mummy?" Dad said. "I know she'll want to see you guys unwrap them in front of her." My brother quickly agreed and started to load the presents into a bag. I, on the other hand, couldn't move. Again, I began to think of my mother. *This will be the last time she'll ever watch us open gifts on Christmas morning.* As if reading my mind, my father put his hand on my face and whispered, "I know, Melin...I know."

I had just about finished getting ready to leave for the hospital when Dad called upstairs to me. "Melinda! Mum's on the phone...do you want to wish her a Merry Christmas?" For the second time in just under an hour, I was rendered motionless. Knowing the anguish that I had undergone having learned of her grim diagnosis, I could only imagine how she must have been feeling. She was the one who was dying. What could I possibly say to her? "Melin?" my dad called again. "Yeah, I'll grab it up here," I said, as I entered my parents' room. I sat down on the left-hand side of their bed, Mum's side, and reluctantly picked up the phone. As I lifted it toward my ear, I wondered what I would possibly say to her. *Just say Merry Christmas and act normally...you can't even imagine what she's going through right now...you need to be strong for her.* "Mum?" I asked, in a timid but controlled manner. The voice I heard on the other end was not the one I'd been expecting. It was filled with joy. "Merry Christmas, Pumpkin!!" my mother said with enthusiasm. For an instant, my heart swelled with happiness, as this was the familiar and cheerful voice I had always known. This was the woman I had always loved; full of life. It was as if nothing had changed. My excitement disappeared as quickly as it came, however, when my father's words came echoing back into my mind. *Three weeks.* This was the last time I would ever speak to my mother on Christmas morning. I felt my face heat up almost instantly, a hallmark sign that I was about to cry. The lump in my throat was sickening, and barely allowed me to breathe. *Don't do it, Melin, don't do it!!!* I was clearly about to lose it on the phone. I felt that if I opened my mouth to speak, I would break down completely. "Melin?" Mum called from the other end of the line. "Are you there, Sweetie?" I was trying my best not to burst into tears. My throat was now completely tightened up and I was holding my breath in an effort to not start bawling. Somehow a few slight whimpers slipped out under my breath. I just hoped Mum didn't hear them. I didn't want to upset her any further. Then, as if she could see what I was going through, my mother spoke. "It's ok, sweetheart. It's ok." It was as if she was there, comforting me through the worst moment of my life. I could all but feel her hands on my face, cooling me down. Mustering up the little composure I had left, I finally uttered the only words I could manage. "I've gotta go, Mum. I'll see you in a little while." Tears consumed me before the phone even reached the receiver. I buried my head in Mum's pillow and wept harder than I'd ever wept in my life. Her scent was still there. I couldn't bear the fact that she would never sleep there again, or that this pillow would eventually lose this beautiful smell. My world was crashing in around me, and I felt like I wanted to die.

Making sure no one saw or heard my emotional collapse, I finally gathered myself enough to get into the car and head to the hospital to see Mum. I breathed an enormous sigh of relief when I saw her. She looked wonderful; the same huge smile, the same loving eyes that disappeared into slits when she laughed. Thankfully, her medication had been adjusted and seemed to have none of the debilitating effects we'd recently witnessed. She was in great spirits. Despite knowing what I did, her demeanor relaxed me. The entire family was there to exchange presents. My brothers and I were pathetic gift-givers, but we gave with the greatest intentions. That year, I'd gotten Mum a squishy reindeer doll to keep her company when we weren't visiting her, and a random tape cassette of Irish music for the boom box she kept in her room. You would have thought I'd given her a diamond necklace and earrings. She couldn't stop thanking me and telling me how much she loved what I'd given her.

After Jimmy and Matt gave her their own CVS-purchased offerings, Mum presented us with our gifts. Because she hadn't been home since before she'd gone to Vegas, my mother understandably hadn't a chance to shop for us. So she improvised. Mum made goody bags out of things she had "collected" from the hospital. Our plastic white bags were filled with Shasta miniature sodas, containers of pudding, hospital sheets and scrubs. Dad's bag had a stethoscope in it. Considering the news we'd all received in the past twenty-four hours, none of us dared make fun of Mum's efforts. She did the best with what she had, right? *This is probably a good time to mention that my mother was a notorious kleptomaniac. A small-scale klepto, but a klepto nonetheless. Hospitals were her playground. She'd steal sodas, canned food, scrubs, johnnies, sheets, pens...anything she could get her hands on. Our beds at home were typically covered in sheets from Mass General. Although*

I'm pretty grossed out thinking about it now, it was hilarious to me at the time. What's even more disturbing is that she was hospitalized as often as she was to enable her to confiscate as much as she did. Mum certainly made the most of it, though. She didn't limit her resource pool to hospitals, however. Our home was filled with ashtrays and salt and pepper shakers from every restaurant at which we'd dined, shampoos and soaps from every hotel we'd ever visited. She was the master. So her gifts to us that Christmas morning could not have been more fitting. Still, keeping the current situation in mind, we started to politely thank Mum for her thoughtfulness. Just as she had mocked our feigned etiquette toward that horrendous pasta dish she'd made during Hurricane Bob, she laughed equally as hard at our attempt of taking her gifts seriously. My mother's uncontrolled laughter was intoxicating, and opened the door for all of us to crack up equally as much. It was so typical of her to do something like that; first to steal, then to make light of possibly the gravest situation imaginable. I was indebted to Mum for so many things, but for her ability to elicit humor in practically any circumstance, especially that morning, I was immeasurably grateful. Several times throughout that visit, I found myself staring at my mother. Her spirits seemed higher than ever, and she actually looked healthier than I'd seen her in weeks. Gazing at her, I just couldn't believe that she'd be gone in less than a month. She was sitting right in front of me. Telling stories. Belly laughing. It just didn't seem possible. Yet my mother made that Christmas magical for everyone. Not with expensive new gifts or decorations or music or games. She saved all of us that day, by allowing us to forget, if only temporarily, what we all knew. Her selflessness and bravery were transcendent.

CHAPTER 18

The Greatest Conversations of My Life

SOME PEOPLE, IF THEY'RE EXTREMELY LUCKY, HAVE THE RARE EXPERIENCE of conversing with another human being on a level of total connectedness and understanding; and in doing so achieve meaning, clarity, and true enlightenment. Most of those select individuals, however, do not experience this level of communication at the age of fourteen.

How many times have you heard someone say, "I wish I had him back for one more day, so I could tell him how much I loved him," or "I hope she realized how much I cared for her?" If there was one good thing about learning of my mother's terminal illness, it was the opportunity I took to have these conversations with her; conversations that most people don't take advantage of having with loved ones, even if given an entire lifetime. I thought of how many people I knew, including Mum, who had lost a parent or a loved one suddenly, without having had the opportunity to say a proper goodbye, or without being able to express their true feelings toward that individual. As evident with my mother when she lost her own father, the inability to convey such emotions or have such conversations can be haunting, and have potentially lasting effects on one's ability to accept or find any sense of peace within death. Also, because it is human nature to think that there will "always be tomorrow," we assume we have unlimited time to ask the questions we've always wanted to ask, or talk candidly about the things that truly matter. This was no longer the case for me. I had three weeks. Three weeks to spend with my dear friend; to ask her everything I had ever wanted to know or wondered, to challenge her, to laugh with her, to cry with her, to let her know exactly how much she meant to me. It was a blessing. Knowing her time was very limited, Mum made it a point to spend quality time with each of her children individually. It was during the time I spent privately with my mother, during the final days of her life, that I experienced the greatest conversations of mine. The following is just a portion of those discussions.

"Are you scared?" I asked. A blunt lead in, perhaps, but it was the first thing that came to mind when I finally sat alone with her. "A little bit," Mum said. "But I'm ready, Sweetie. It's just my time. I fought this thing as best I could, and I'm not giving up. My body has just given out. I've experienced so many emotions during the past three years. At first I was very hopeful, then frustrated, then angry, then hopeful again...I've run the gamut. And I'm tired. It took me a while but I've come to terms with the fact that we've done everything we can...that's humanly possible anyway." She paused for a moment. "Now it's in God's hands. He clearly has a plan for me. It's different from the one I'd imagined, but I've come to accept it. Do I wish I could have more time with you and your brothers and your father? Of course I do, Sweetie. Was I pissed when I found out? Initially, yes. But I always knew this was a possibility. So now I have a choice: I can either be bitter at the world or I can come to peace with myself and my life. I've asked myself the tough questions, and I've come to realize that it's not how *long* you live your life, it's how *well* you live it. Have I lived a good life? Have I been a good person? Have I treated others with kindness and decency? Am I leaving this world a better place? The answer to all of these questions is yes, and that's all that really matters now. It's really that simple, Babe. I take my dying young as God's way of telling me that I've accomplished everything I was intended to...I just happened to do it in forty-four years. So if you look at it that way, I'm an overachiever...most of the old bastards on this floor have taken twice as long to do their jobs!" She smiled. "I now realize that this *(she lifted her hands to her chest, implying her physical being)* is just temporary. That's all it is. We all eventually go home. That's why I'm not scared anymore."

"When you say, 'home,' do you mean Heaven? Do you believe in Heaven?" I asked. "Yes, very much," my mother answered. "Not in the way I used to, though. When we're young, we tend to understand things on a very simplified scale; partially because we have a limited capacity to comprehend complexity, and also because we are taught by others to view things in such a manner. It's a necessary evil to a certain extent. For example, when I was a little girl I believed in the stereotypical notion of Heaven: white, fluffy clouds, St. Peter in front the pearly gates. This is the vision most Catholics are given by their parents or teachers. It's a picture that is painted for us to convey a point: that if we live our lives in a manner which God sees fit, then we will be rewarded. We will get to live eternally in Paradise. It's a metaphor. Much of what we learn as children is not meant to be taken literally but is, because it's all we're capable of at the time. Since I've grown older, and specifically since I've been ill, I've reevaluated most everything in my life, including some very fundamental issues such as God, religion, and the afterlife. I guess the closer you are to death, the more you want to understand life; its purpose, our purpose within it, what it all means in the grand scale of things. Is this all there is? There are plenty of people who will never venture to ask themselves these questions; in part because of close-mindedness, or perhaps they're terrified of what they might discover. On the other hand, I *had* to know. I had to differentiate between that which I had been taught and that which I genuinely believed. I believe Heaven is an elevated state of existence and consciousness; a nonphysical place where our souls reside after leaving our bodies. Your soul is your essence; it is what makes you who you are. It is bound by nothing. It's difficult to grasp, because you've only known me as this: what you see in front of your eyes. But what makes me who I truly am: my spirit, my energy, my character…is not what you're looking at right now. It's inside. It's who's been your mother for the past fourteen years. It's who loves you more than anything else in the world. It's not this *(again, she raised her hands to her chest)*. Your body is just a package which houses your soul for a given amount of time here on earth. Eventually, the package wears down but what's inside does not. So when I die, I'm not really going anywhere, Sweetheart. My soul is just being liberated by my body, kind of like a butterfly when it breaks free of its cocoon. I'll be in a different form, but I will be here nonetheless. Do you understand?" "Yes," I replied. I'd never thought of Heaven or death in this way.

She continued. "It's going to be a challenge for you, Babe, to adjust to that. It's always hard to view things in a different light than that in which you've always known them. It's simple to believe in things you can see and touch and feel. But for you to truly trust in what I'm saying, you'll have to go beyond your bodily senses. You'll have to engage your faith. Faith is the sense of the soul. Only in it will you find truth in what I've told you. Once you have the ability to transcend the physical and understand things on an authentic level, you'll find enlightenment. That, in itself, is heavenly."

Mum's words were immeasurably comforting. For the first time, I realized that my relationship with her didn't have to end with her death. I could keep her with me. Then I started to think about those who would never get a chance to know her. "You're never going to get a chance to meet my husband or my children, though," I said in sadness. "They will never have an opportunity to know you as I do." My mother smiled gently, and her eyes filled with tears. "Maybe not exactly as you do," she said, "but they can come to know me through you. Talk to them about me, tell stories about me, laugh about me, cry about me. That's the only way they'll ever get to know me. Will you do me that honor?" I nodded my head and began to cry. "Don't ever be sad when you speak of me, Pumpkin," Mum said. "It's in doing so that you will enable me to continue living…so keep me with you. When you go off to college and when you fall in love, when you get married and when you have your children…keep me with you. As long as I'm in your mind and your heart, I will never miss a single moment."

By mentioning marriage and children, my mother raised one of the issues I had only recently begun to ponder. At fourteen, I had just started to express interest in dating. While most people were well aware of my tomboyishness, very few knew that I was tremendously sentimental when it came to the idea of love. Since I was a little girl I dreamt of finding the man whose love would beautify my life; the soul who could see into mine. Although I'd always fantasized about meeting this person, I had absolutely no clue as to how I would discover him or recognize him when he came into my life. "How will I know when I'm truly in love? How will I know when I've met the person I'm supposed to marry?" I asked my mother in a hopeful tone. Mum's entire expression changed with this inquiry. Though she would have answered a thousand more questions regarding life and death, I think she was delighted I changed the subject. "You're probably not going to be satisfied with my answer, mainly because you won't be able to fully appreciate it until you experience what I'm about to say. As cliché as it sounds, you will just know. I know that's not the answer you are looking for, but it's true. You'll feel it in the very depths of your soul. You'll feel it in your bones. When you fall in love it will be forever, Babe. I don't see you falling in love too many times in your life. Not because you're not worthy or capable, but because you already know what you want. You've never been the type of girl who simply wants to get married for the sake of getting married. You're looking for the real thing—to fall madly in love, to find your other half, the person who truly challenges you and completes you. You want true love, in the deepest sense of the word. So although you'll meet plenty of men in your life, many of whom will be great guys, you will not pursue them past a certain point if you don't see it leading to that standard. That's the way it should be. Don't negotiate your passion or ideals. For the right man, you won't have to. He will respect you and love you and understand you on a level which few others ever will. You'll share a love so deep that it will be apparent to all who know you. And it will be the most natural and beautiful feeling on earth. That's what I mean when I say 'you'll just know.' It will be like nothing you've ever felt before, and at the same time will be the most organic thing you've ever experienced. A huge part of finding what you want is realizing what you don't want. There may be times when you think you're in love, or that you've met the right guy, but if you need to question yourself about it then you'll know it's not the case. So even though you might have your heart broken by a few people along the way, you'll be better off for it. Every experience, good or bad, is an opportunity to learn more about yourself and what will truly make you happy. Trust your heart. There are plenty of things in life on which you can compromise, Honey, but not in this department. Love has always been the most important thing in your life, and that's never going to change, so don't ever settle for less than what you've always imagined. Your husband will be your angel, and you, his. There is nothing in this world more worthy of waiting for, so be patient. He'll come into your life when you least expect it." Although I would have liked a more definitive answer, Mum's explanation inspired me, and made sense to me on a very core level. The more she spoke, the more I realized how well she knew me, which is why I trusted her words.

At the same time, it was agonizing for me to think that this woman, who clearly understood me better than anyone, would be gone in a few weeks. My best friend was dying. While I felt strengthened by my mother's wisdom, I had yet to completely absorb it, so my vulnerability remained. My heart ached at the thought of losing her. "What are we going to do without you, Mum?" I whispered, as I felt a familiar warmth stream down my face. My mother reached for me. "Come here, Sweetheart." She shifted over in her hospital bed and pulled me in closely. As I nestled into her, I was instantly transported to safety. Closing my eyes, I returned to my favorite childhood nightly ritual of Mum's tucking me into bed. For as long as I could remember, I fell asleep to the gentleness of my mother's voice and hands. Every night at bedtime, she'd either sit or lie beside me and talk quietly while rubbing my head, back, and bum until I slipped into a blissful state of hibernation. *Without reservation, I credit my ability to fall asleep virtually anywhere at anytime to my mum, who made falling asleep one of my favorite things in life.* For a moment there was no cancer, there was no pain. There was only mother and daughter. I didn't want to open my eyes. This dream was too sacred to leave behind. "I'm not worried about you, Melin." Mum's voice brought me back to reality. "I know you'll be fine. You're strong and you have such a good heart, Sweetie. As long as you continue to listen to it then you'll always be ok. You're intelligent and passionate and emotional…you have a very good balance in life. Don't try to be perfect all the time. I know it's in your nature but keep things in perspective. Remember what's important. The only expectations you should be concerned with meeting or surpassing are your own. Don't ever change who you are to meet someone else's mold. Maintain your individuality. Vigorously pursue your dreams, and don't be afraid of failure. Your heart was built not to wonder, but to believe. So go after everything you ever want in life. You deserve it. Keep a clear and open mind. Realize that certain people's opinions are the result of their upbringing, and not their true feelings. Your father and I have undoubtedly made comments in front of you and your brothers that were in poor taste. Although we meant no harm, we were still wrong. Be color-blind. Don't adopt prejudice. Give everyone in life an equal chance. Treat every person you meet exactly the way you'd like to be treated…with kindness, fairness, and respect. When it comes down to it, that's what God wants of us; to treat each other with love and decency and to live our lives in a manner that reflects Him. That's it. Don't get caught up in ritual or formality. While we are all guilty of this to some degree, don't let it control you. Always remember fundamental purpose. Think freely and keep your mind active. Take nothing or no one for granted. Don't ever pass up an opportunity to tell those you care about exactly how you feel about them. You never know if you'll get another chance. As trivial as it may seem, if you have something nice to say, *say it*. Don't hold back. The same goes with that smile of yours. Never stop sharing it with others. It may mean more to someone than you'll ever know. Recognize angels in your life, for as you will be blessed *with* them, you will also *be* one to someone else. Don't ration your love. It's the one resource on this earth that I'm convinced is infinite. Don't ever be ashamed to cry, whether in sadness or in joy. There are few physical acts more genuine than this. Continue to wear your heart on your sleeve. Your unpretentiousness is what draws people to you. And never forget to laugh at yourself, Sweetie. Don't ever take yourself or life too seriously. It's too short not to enjoy, so embrace it, as you've already started to do." My mother spoke with an assuredness I'd seen in few others. Her confidence was infectious, her words were invigorating. For the first time, I started to believe that I would be ok.

"Dad and your brothers are going to be alright, too, Melin," Mum continued. "You're all going to have to come together and help each other, though. There will be plenty of people you'll meet in life; acquaintances and friends will come and go, but your family will always be there. They are your blood, your very lifeline, and you will need to stay close and take care of one another. Your father is a unique soul. He's one of the strongest men I've ever met, yet one of the most sensitive. He's going to need you, Sweetie. You've always been his little girl…be his friend as well. Keep him involved in your life. Let him know how much you love him. And don't be afraid to put him in his place if he needs to be. He's set in his ways but don't let him get trapped in them. Challenge him. Believe me, he'll be better for it. Don't feel that you'll have to play housewife just because you'll be the only female in the house. All the responsibilities will have to be split up equally. Everyone is going to need to do his share. Your brother Jimmy is going to need to reconnect with all of you when he comes home. It's not going to be easy for him. He's been through a lot, Babe, more than any of us will ever understand. Watch out for him. He's one of the most trusting, gentle people you'll ever know, and has so much to give. He's just a little lost right now. He'll find his way, I have no doubt. Just give him your love and support. Be his friend. That alone will help him get where he needs to be. And then there's Matt, my Baby Bud. I can already see it; you are going to be inseparable. Take care of him, Melin. You don't have to be his mother, but take care of him. He's going to need you more than anyone. Whether you expect it or not, he will look to you for guidance. Matt has a great heart and a wonderful spirit; help him nurture them. In a way, I'm thankful that he doesn't fully understand what's going on right now. I think it would be too much for him to handle at such a young age. But when he does realize it, I'll be gone, and it will affect him deeply. You need to be there for him. As emotional as he is, he keeps everything inside. Be his outlet. He'll be yours for the rest of your life, so look out for one another." My mother paused, and lifted my chin with her hand, bringing my eyes directly to hers. All I could see was love. "You'll all be fine. Trust me, Sweetie," she whispered. My heart swelled as I felt Mum's lips press against my forehead. I believed her. There, lying in my mother's arms, I found peace.

CHAPTER 19

Goodbye

"WHAT ARE THEY GOING TO DO, PUT ME IN THE CORNER?" THIS WAS MY mum's response when we caught her smoking in her hospital room bathroom, a week before she died. Bold to her last breath. New Year's had come and gone, and my mother's condition had taken its final turn. Although heavily medicated, she was completely perceptive the last time I saw her, which was four days before her death. I had a basketball game scheduled at school that night. Lately, my father had been encouraging me to go to more of my games and practices, as we'd been spending so much time in the hospital. He felt sports were a good form of release and distraction for me. That particular night, however, he told me I'd better come into Boston to see Mum. While I never thought it would be the last opportunity I'd have with her, I knew those three weeks were almost finished. That final visit was as normal and relaxed as any I'd had with her. Mum was very much herself; laughing and joking, making obscene gestures with the squishy reindeer I bought her for Christmas. She was relentless with her humor. Most of all, my mother seemed very calm, which was evident in her playfulness. When it was time to leave, I hugged and kissed her as I always did. "I love you Mum, I'll see you soon," I said, as I wrapped my arms around her. As I pulled away, I felt her draw me back in, not wanting to let go. I reestablished my embrace, and positioned myself closer to her so I could hold onto her more tightly. *Don't let her go until she lets you go,* I silently promised myself. We must have gone through the same routine about five more times before I finally left. Had I known it would be the last time, I'm not quite sure if I ever would have let go. As my father walked me out of the room, I kept turning back to see my mother. "I love you Mum," I kept saying, as if she didn't hear me. Finally, she slipped out of sight behind the door. After two brief steps down the hall, I sneaked under Dad's arm and back into her doorway. "I love you Mum." She was sitting up in bed, covered comfortably to her waist in blankets, with her feet crossed casually and her head propped up with pillows. It was the last time I would see my mother alive. She looked peaceful, and happy. With a radiant smile, Mum spoke her final words to me, "I love you, Sweetheart." She blew a kiss and waved to me as I backed away from her room. It was a familiar sight, but with new meaning.

"*...wave to them. Those are your angels waving down to you from Heaven.*"

After that night, my mother required a progressively increasing level of medication, which gradually diminished her consciousness. Because Mum wanted me and my brothers to remember her in complete clarity, she requested that only my father come to see her from that point forward. My Aunt Mary stayed at the house with Matt and me, as Dad was now sleeping overnight in the hospital with Mum. The night before she died, I was home studying for a literature test. <u>Great</u> <u>Expectations</u> by Charles Dickens. As much as I adored the book, I couldn't concentrate. My mind was overworked with emotion. Finally, when my brain was fried, I asked my little brother to test me on the material. He started goofing around and I quickly became annoyed with him. Whether my frustration was fueled by my complete lack of knowledge retention, or Matt's silliness when I was trying to focus, it mattered not. I simply erupted. My rage was so intense I nearly struck my brother. I yelled so loud and so hard at him that I could actually feel the veins pulsing out of my neck. It was senseless and completely unfounded, but I just needed to scream. My poor aunt ran upstairs to see what all the commotion was. I pushed past her in the hallway and locked myself in the bathroom, nearly putting a hole in the door as I pounded it shut. For nearly five minutes, I went into a rampage; shouting at the top of my lungs, banging on the countertops and kicking the linen closet door. Eventually, with my fists and feet throbbing in self-induced pain, I began to cry. I was exhausted, in every sense of the word. Suddenly I heard a gentle knock on the door. "Melinda-bird? Will you let me in, Honey?" Aunt Mary had waited calmly outside the bathroom while I threw my fit. I was ashamed of myself. My mum's oldest sister, a nun, had just overheard me bellow out some of the worst profanities in the English language, yet she was still speaking delicately to me. Out of respect, I gathered myself and embarrassingly opened the door. "Sorry Aunt Mare," I began to say, my head hanging in shame. She interrupted before I could finish my sentence. "Nothing to apologize for, Sweetie...nothing at all," she said as she wrapped her arms around me. Until that point in my life, I hadn't had a particularly strong kinship with my aunt. At that moment though, I felt closer to her than almost anyone. I thanked God for her empathy. Instantly, I felt understood. "You're not going to believe this, but I had a very similar outburst not even six hours ago when you guys were in school," she confessed. Looking at her in disbelief, I questioned whether she'd be capable of such outrage. "You?!" I asked. "Well, you probably gave the doors and counters a better beating than I did, but I did my best," she said grinning. "The screaming and swearing were dead-on matches, though." I couldn't believe what I was hearing. She continued, "I haven't worn a habit in years, Honey. I've been working with recovering alcoholics and drug addicts and prisoners for most of my life. I've heard it all." Her honesty and humor were healing. "Earlier today, I was in here putting towels away. I'd noticed the laundry had been piling up and I wanted to get a few loads done for you kids and your Dad. As I placed the linens in the closet, I looked at the towels that your mother had folded and realized I hadn't folded them in the same way. I tried for about twenty minutes to get them to look as good as hers but I just couldn't, and before I knew it I'd ripped every damn face cloth and hand cloth out of that closet, threw them on the ground, then plopped down on them and began to cry." I looked at her and realized that we were more similar than I'd previously thought. "It seems stupid, I know, but I think we both understand that I wasn't upset about the towels," my aunt explained. "I was just so sad thinking about your mother dying. She's one of my favorite people in the whole world. Your mum has been such a positive force in my life. She's never judged me, and has been one of my best friends. And the thought of losing her just sucks. So my sorrow manifested itself in anger and it got the best of me. It happens to the best of us, Melin. And you know what? It's ok. Everyone needs to let off steam sometimes. It's better to take it out on objects rather than people, right?" She smiled as she walked over to the closet. Opening the door, she said, "You know what the best part is? In the middle of my crying fit, I heard your mother's voice. *What the hell are you doing you crazy old nun?!? Have some pride...you're weeping in a pile of laundry! Get your ass up and fold those towels!*" With my hand to God,

I swear I heard her clear as day, in that wisecracking tone. I almost wet myself laughing thinking about how silly I looked. So I did as she said; I picked my butt up off the floor, folded those towels, and went on with my day. I'm not angry with myself for breaking down, I'm just so thankful that your mother was there to pick me up, even though she wasn't here physically."

That was the first time I'd heard my mother spoken of in such a manner; as if she were an angel. As I listened to my aunt's story, I realized that she had saved me every bit as much as my mum had saved her earlier that day. My mother's words resonated in my mind. *God sends angels in many forms.*

CHAPTER 20

Snow

JANUARY 13, 1993. AFTER A LONG NIGHT OF LAUGHING AND CRYING WITH my aunt, I woke up early to restudy for my test. It was snowing. I immediately turned on the television to see if school had been cancelled. To my dismay, it had not. Eventually, Matt and Aunt Mary joined me downstairs. "How are you getting to school today, Melin?" she asked me. "It's your turn to drive today," I told her. While my brother, still in junior high, took the bus to school, I carpooled to Cardinal Spellman in Brockton, which was two towns away, with two other kids from my hometown. Since we were only freshmen, our parents would rotate driving schedules. "Oh, no," she responded. "Not in this stuff. You know I don't drive in snow. You're going to have to get one of the other parents to drive." I had forgotten about my aunt's driving phobias.

No rain. No snow. No darkness. *Damn*, I thought, as I didn't want to inconvenience the other parties. Unfortunately, after calling the two other households to explain the situation, neither of them could make it across town to pick me up, as the weather had grown progressively worse. Normally, facing the possibility of missing a day of school and a test would have caused me to panic, but my exhaustion dominated any potential guilt. Initially not knowing what to do with myself, I sat down on the couch and started flipping through the channels on TV. Stopping eventually at VH1, I decided to lie down with the intention of closing my eyes for only a few minutes. But the warmth of the house and the soft light of the snow-filled sky on my face were hypnotizing. I started to drift into sleep. The lyrics of the video I was watching became part of my dream. *"I will be walking one day, down a street far away, and see a face in the crowd, and smile. Knowing how you made me laugh. Hearing sweet echoes of you from the past. I will remember you."* The song was "I Will Remember You," by Amy Grant. It was the last thing I remember before my father woke me.

I returned to consciousness in a very peaceful manner, to the sensation of my feet being rubbed. At first, I thought our cat may have been snuggling up against them, as she often did. When I finally had my bearings, I realized it was my father, sitting at the end of the couch, who'd delicately awoken me. When he came into clear sight, there was a look on his face that I'd never seen before. "Hey Pumpkin," he said gently. His voice was uncharacteristically softened, and although he wasn't crying, his face was worn with tears. I hadn't seen him in three days, and it seemed as if he hadn't slept since. Dad became tight-lipped and put his head down almost immediately, as if to avoid any chance of my seeing him break down. I wanted nothing more than to go back to sleep and wake up to realize that this was only a dream; that my father wouldn't tell me what I knew he was about to tell me. "Sit up Melin," he said in a broken voice. I sat up and positioned myself directly beside him, so we were joined at the hip. I could not bear to look at him, as I could physically hear him choking on his own tears. But my sympathy for him forced me to raise my eyes to his. I couldn't breathe. Dad finally took my hand in his and gathered the only strength he had left to speak. His voice cracked in agony. "Mummy died, sweetie." My father, who I'd never seen cry fully, began to weep. He grabbed me and pulled me into him. "She's in Heaven now," he said through his sobbing. I went numb. *This isn't real*, I told myself. *This can't be happening*. With my arms wrapped tightly around him, I felt Dad's shoulders shaking up and down in convulsions. That's when I lost it. I buried my head in his chest and cried uncontrollably for what seemed like an eternity. "She's not in pain anymore, Melin. No more pain," my father whispered, as he stroked the back of my head. While these words would have normally provided me with some sense of solace, I was overtaken with the most excruciating grief I'd ever known. I was inconsolable for a brief while, but the thought of my father's own sorrow eventually impelled me to gather myself. When there were no more tears left to cry, I asked him, "How did she die? Was she in pain?" With a deep sigh, my father walked me through Mum's final hours. "No, she wasn't in pain. The morning after you saw her, she started getting really sick, which required her to be heavily medicated. Her lungs were filled with fluid so the doctors removed it with a needle, which was very painful. Although she was virtually in a coma at that point, and may not have been able to feel it, I didn't want her to go through any more suffering, so I decided against having the procedure repeated when her lungs filled up again. Late last night, the doctor told me to get in touch with whomever I needed to, because he did not expect her to make it through the morning. I contacted all of your aunts and they planned on heading in this morning. When I saw the weather, though, I called them all back and told them not to come, that it was too dangerous. So it was just me and her in the end. It was very peaceful, like she was sleeping.

I just held her hand and watched her. Slowly her breaths grew further and further apart, until finally she took one last deep breath, and then she was gone. Her head nodded gently down into her chest…and she was gone. She went very peacefully." As my father described my mother's passing, I recalled the visions she had shared with me just a week earlier. She had compared her soul leaving her body to a butterfly leaving its cocoon. It sounded as if her body released her soul with that final breath. I wondered where she was flying just then. Knowing my mother was no longer encapsulated with pain gave me great comfort. In the same right, the challenge which Mum predicted I would face was beginning. My faith would undoubtedly be tested. I'd listened to her notions of Heaven and death and the soul, and found great peace within her words. But now that she was "gone," could I truly believe what she told me? Could I practice what she preached? As my mind started to race, my father's voice brought me back to reality. Taking my face in his hands, he asked "Are you ok, Pumpkin?" with pure emotion in his eyes. Although still extremely distraught, he had stopped crying and was now focused only on consoling me. Looking at my father, I tried to imagine how difficult the past few hours had been for him. I couldn't fathom how heartbreaking it must have been for him to have watched my mother die. As peaceful as it may have been, he saw the love of his life take her last breath. There was absolutely nothing I could think of that could possibly be more devastating. But yet here he was, selflessly taking care of me. He was never more a father than he was in that moment. Without saying a word, I nodded my head and embraced him again. For so many reasons up to that point in my life, my dad had been the strongest person in the world to me. But this single occasion redefined my understanding of his strength, and made me love my father more than I already had, which I didn't think was possible.

Shortly thereafter, Dad and I picked up Matt at school. When we arrived, my father went to the principal's office to tell them the news, while I went upstairs to get my brother. On my way, I passed my former janitor who was cheerful to see me. "Hey Melin!!!" he said with excitement. "What are you doing back here? How's everything going?" Mr. G. was a great guy, and someone with whom I'd always stop and talk when I'd gone to school there. However, on this day I knew I couldn't even look at him without bursting into tears. "Fine," I said quickly as I lowered my head and rushed quickly past him. As much as I tried not to, I began to cry. I ran up the stairs before he could ask why. When I reached the third floor, I stopped to collect myself. Wiping my face dry, I took a deep breath and thought of what I was going to say to Matt. Before I could find the words, my brother's best friend Jay, who'd been standing in the hallway and spotted me through the glass doors, started walking toward me. "Hey Melin! Playin' hookie today?" he joked. As he reached me, his demeanor changed instantly. Jay was like a brother to me, and was extremely close to my entire family, including my mum. He had been well aware of the severity of her condition. Despite my best efforts, my eyes started to well up again. "Oh no," he said. Always an emotionally intelligent kid, Jay instinctively put his arms around me. There was no fighting it. I began to weep on his shoulder as he hugged me. In turn, he also began to cry intensely. "I'm so sorry," he kept saying as we held each other. Wiping my eyes, I saw my brother walk out of the bathroom and into the hallway where Jay and I were standing. He froze. Unbeknownst to me, while he was in the restroom, he had seen me and my father pull up to the school. Despite his naïveté regarding the terminality of my mother's illness, he knew why we were there. Seeing Jay and I confirmed it for him. Before Matt could say anything, I grabbed him and embraced him. As I continued to cry, I whispered brokenly into his ear, "Mum died, Matt." My brother was silent. He held on to me tightly as he absorbed my words. At that point, Jay had joined us and wrapped his arms around Matt and me. As his best friend and I wept, my little brother almost didn't react at all. His eyes filled up but he didn't really cry. He was in shock. I'd feared this moment. While I had been somewhat thankful for his unknowingness to that point, I knew it would make that moment much more difficult when it arrived. We eventually gathered his things and met Dad downstairs. The devastation of my mother's death rendered my brother speechless for much of the remainder of the day.

The rest of the afternoon was a blur. My aunts were at the house when we arrived home. Sally and Mary stayed with my father to help him with the funeral arrangements, while Eileen and Peggy took Matt and me to the mall. Initially, I thought they'd taken us there to take our minds off the events of the morning, but in fact they'd done so to buy us proper attire for the upcoming services. When we returned home, we were greeted at the door by my high school chaplain, Father Al Faretra. He was a lovely man, of whom I had quickly become fond in the short time I knew him. One of the kindest people I'd ever met, Fr. Al had come to the house to assist my Dad. For my father's sake, I was grateful that so many people were there. I couldn't bear the thought of his having to handle those details by himself.

Dusk was coming. Although thankful for the company, I needed to be alone. I went upstairs to my bedroom and closed the door, strangely relieved by my solitude. Kneeling on my bed, I cranked open the windows and felt winter's breath on my face. It was invigorating. Inhaling deeply, I smelled the aroma of my neighbor's wood-burning fire. As my lungs filled with ice-cold fresh air, I felt cleansed. I sat down cross-legged in my bed and stared into the approaching night. Background noise soon faded as I became enraptured in the utter silence of the evening. It was the sort of absolute stillness that only a snowfall can bring. The flakes, now reflecting a light shade of blue, had gathered beautifully on the landscape. Like my mother, I had always been captivated by the ability of snow to make ordinary scenery seem magical. While I looked upon this peaceful spectacle, I tried to grasp the idea that my mother was no longer on this earth. It was difficult to conceptualize. Gazing outward, I saw pure physical beauty. Though my senses were engorged by things I could see and smell and feel, the one thing I wanted wasn't there. I couldn't see her. I couldn't hug her. I couldn't smell her gorgeous scent. My mother was gone. For what seemed like the hundredth time that day, I began to cry. I'd never felt so lonely. As hollowness began to overtake me, I was stimulated by a bone-chilling breeze which rushed through my window. As sure as I'd been of anything in my life, I felt my mum in that moment. The cold air on my face felt uncannily reminiscent. One of my favorite feelings in the world was when my mother would blow on my face when I was crying. It would instantly cool me down. It was one of the many little things she did which made a huge difference. In recalling her kindnesses, I viewed my mother's idiosyncrasies in a different light than I ever had before. They were no longer simply things that she did that were uniquely her. They *were* her. They made her who she was. And they were now sacred. As this subtle revelation came over me, my mother's words echoed in my memory. *I'll be with you every bit as much as I am now, Sweetie. You won't be able to see me, but you'll feel me.* For the first time, I began to truly comprehend what Mum was trying to convey. I felt it in my soul. She was there with me. This moment, which has remained private to me until now, was quietly one of the happiest of my life. It was the birth of my spirituality. Lying down to sleep, I looked upon an onyx sky, and saw a few lingering snowflakes make their way down to my windowsill. *Souvenirs,* I thought, as I gazed upwardly, grinning. While she may not have been there rubbing my back or my head or my bum, my mother, nonetheless, tucked me in to bed that night.

CHAPTER 21

Whirlwind

Mum passed away on a Wednesday, and her services began that Friday. She was waked for two full days and nights. Four wakes in total. Anything less would have been inadequate. Though I'd only attended one previous wake, my grandfather's, I realized that my mother's was inordinately packed. For two straight afternoons and evenings, the funeral home was filled with people who had come to pay their respects to my mum. Immediate family, distant relatives, friends, acquaintances, and those who knew her only by association lined up for hours to say their final goodbyes. Every wake ran late, due to an overflow of attendees. Though I was overwhelmed by such a tribute, I was dazed with emotion. The entire experience was very surreal. My father, my brothers, and I stood for hours in a receiving line, greeting hundreds of mourners. People whom I didn't even know would grab me and hug me and tell me how much I meant to my mother, and how much she meant to them. Others would burst into tears at the sight of us, telling us how tragic it was for us to have lost Mum at such a young age. And then there were those who would pray silently at her casket, and quietly share their condolences with us. Though I appreciated all of the sentiments that were expressed to me, I cannot accurately recall much of what was said due to the bewilderment of the situation. The entire scene seemed illusory. In between the whirlwind of well wishes and sympathies, I would periodically look over at my mother's body. While at first I avoided the sight, I eventually became captivated by it. The longer I looked at her, the more I realized she wasn't there. It was as she'd said when she referred to the body as a shell; it remained though she was gone. Even still, I could not take my eyes off of her.

In the midst of my surroundings, I often fell into daydreams. I wondered what Mum would have thought of these affairs. In one right, I thought she would have been extremely moved by the outpouring of people who had come to pay tribute to her. On the other hand, I bet she would have loved to have had a traditional Irish wake. Mum would have reveled in the idea of her family and friends gathering together over food and drink to toast and celebrate her life. In my opinion, no one was more deserving of such a memorialization. While nearly everyone who knew her felt as if her life ended too early, the way in which she lived it far exceeded anything that could be measured in terms of years. What my mother did with her forty-four years of life on this earth, in and of itself, was cause for celebration, and based on what she'd shared with me in regards to Heaven, the life she was moving onto was cause for celebration also. For those reasons, combined with the fact that Mum turned practically every situation she was involved with into a party, I wished her wakes could have been more joyous, as I'm sure she would have wanted them. Simultaneously, I could not escape the undeniable sorrow I felt deep within my heart. While I tried my best to keep in mind the transcendental qualities of the soul which my mother shared with me, it was difficult not to be consumed by the circumstances.

After the first service, Dad, Jimmy, Matt and I went home for a few hours to unwind before we needed to return that evening. As a form of release, I picked up a pen and started to write. The day before, I'd told my father that I wanted to eulogize my mother. Knowing that my love of words and writing were equally as strong as Mum's, Dad didn't hesitate in granting my request. Considering what I'd experienced in the past few weeks, I had no problem pouring my emotion out on paper. Paying no mind initially to grammar, flow, or organization, I concentrated only on getting my raw thoughts on paper. Start to finish, it took me about an hour to complete. Realizing the element of finality which the pending funeral would bring, but also recognizing the continuity of my mother's life, I was impelled to write about the future. So I wrote a letter to Mum. I penned my work as if she would read it, as I fully intended her to hear it. While I expressed my longing to have her here for all the life events that she would miss, I also shared my belief that she would in fact be here for everything; as long as, as she'd asked, we kept her with us. It was, in many respects, my first prayer to my mother.

The fourth and final wake was held the following night. I'd been welling up with tears the entire evening, but the commotion of people and prayer cards and commiseration kept me from being able to truly absolve. As the ceremony was nearing its close, I was approached by my mother's sister Eileen. She'd always reminded me of Mum. Their looks and sense of humor were frighteningly similar, but their boldness is what made them nearly identical. They were audacious, and while tactful most of the time, neither could be stopped from expressing their opinions or (for lack of a better term) cutting through the bullshit. Sensing my exhaustion, and without saying a word, she gently wrapped her arms around me. We were standing directly in front of my mother's casket. Holding her, I may as well have been embracing my mum. Though I had kept my composure for nearly the entire duration of the services, this unspoken connection prompted me to break down completely. With pure emotion, I wept deeply on my aunt's shoulder. As my bawling intensified, I tucked my head toward her neck to muffle my wailing. Squeezing me tightly, she whispered, "I know, Sweetie. I know." Not once loosening her hold, Aunt Eileen let me cry for as long as I needed. "Let it out, Babe," she encouraged, fully aware of my need to unleash. Eventually, when I finished sobbing and caught my breath, my aunt walked me out of the crowd and found a quiet spot in the hall near the water bubbler. "Sit down, Melin," she said, pouring me a glass. Taking a deep breath, I felt liberated. I was profoundly grateful to Eileen for allowing me to release as I did. Taking the seat beside me, she began to speak. "Honey, I don't know how to sugarcoat this, so I'm just going to say it." In true fashion, she wasted no time with delicacy. Once again, it was like having my mother there. "Right now, you are surrounded by so many people you can't even breathe. While it's a good thing in that you have an overload of love and support from practically everyone you've ever known in your life, that support system will slowly but surely break down over time. There are lots of people you've seen over the past few days who have offered their help and said things like, 'if there's anything I can do' or 'if you ever need anything from me…' Although well-intentioned, they will eventually and naturally fade back into their normal lives while you guys and your father adjust to your new lives without your mum. When the funeral is over tomorrow, and you and your dad and your brothers go home, that's when the silence is going to kick in and it's not going to be easy. I went through it when I lost Peter (her husband, who died at the age of thirty-three of pancreatic cancer). I'm not trying to depress you Sweetie, I'm just leveling with you. If we're lucky, God gives each of us a few key people in our lives on whom we can truly depend and trust." My aunt lifted my chin with her hand. "I will always be here for you, Melin." As she looked into my eyes, I felt my mother speaking to me through her. It was the same voice, the same Irish face, the same squinty blue eyes, thin nose and lips. Looking at her, and holding her hands, I felt the full impact of what she was saying. Without thought, I put my arms around her in appreciation. Although not in the traditional sense of the word, I had just "met" my first angel after having lost my mother. While she had been there my entire life, it was only then that I realized her true identity. To this day, my Aunt Eileen is the closest thing in the world I have to my mum.

CHAPTER 22

Requiem

It was eight o'clock on the morning of my mother's funeral. Although bitterly cold outside, the funeral parlor was warmed with radiant sunshine which poured through the windows. While all other family and friends had paid their final respects and were now waiting in the procession line in the parking lot, only my father, my brothers, and I remained in the reposing room with my mother's body. So far, this was the most difficult moment I'd faced since Mum's death. As the four of us stood in silence in front of her casket, my father began to cry. At first I hesitated to look at him, knowing that doing so would cause me to start sobbing as well. I grabbed him around his waist and hugged him tightly. Dad bellowed deeply as he put his arms around me, and started to weep uncontrollably. With my free arm, I grabbed my brother Jimmy by the shirtsleeve, pulling him toward us. Both he and Matt responded instinctively, and joined us in a unified embrace. Dad squeezed us with all his might. "I love you guys," my father said, as his chest heaved with convulsions. "I love you so much. We have to take care of each other now. That's what Mummy wanted." With the exception of my little brother, who had yet to truly cry, we all bawled our eyes out as we held on to one another. Although I was experiencing one of the saddest moments of my life, I felt comforted by the solidarity of my family. Eventually gathering ourselves, we made our final partings with my mother. Jim and Matt kneeled together and prayed by her side. I followed with my father standing behind me. As I knelt before her, I reached into my pocket and removed a folded, handwritten copy of the eulogy I had composed, and silently read it to her. At points, my tears blinded me from being able to read what I had written. When I finished, I refolded the piece of paper and placed it beside her in the casket. Putting my hand to my lips, I kissed my fingers and placed them on Mum's hands. They were cold as ice. Being the first time I had touched a dead body, I was unprepared for what it felt like. Although slightly shaken by the ordeal, it solidified my belief that my mum was in fact no longer there; that this was in fact, her shell. Even so, I had trouble letting her go. *This is the last time I will lay eyes on you in this life*, I thought, as my throat tightened in agony. It was hard to conceive. Wiping my eyes, I looked upon her face for the last time and stared. "I love you, Mum," I whispered, as I slowly backed away from her body. I joined my brothers in the entryway of the room while my father remained with my mother. Though composed, he was once again consumed with tears. Gazing at him from afar, I felt more sympathy for my father at that moment than I had ever felt for any human being. Leaning down to my mother, Dad spoke more softly and delicately than I'd ever heard him speak. While I would have loved to have known what he'd said to her, his words were inaudible to me. With full intention, his last words to her were private. Finally, he ran his hand over her hair and kissed her gently on the lips. "I love you, Monk," I heard him say, as he pulled himself away from the casket. Dad cried unashamedly as he wrapped his arms around our shoulders and walked us out of the funeral home.

Immaculate Conception Church in Stoughton may have never seen a more packed house. As I sat in the limousine in the church parking lot with my brothers and my Dad, I couldn't believe my eyes. There was a traffic jam at the intersection due to a backup of mourners trying to find parking spaces in a lot that had already been filled to capacity. Eventually, funeral goers lined the surrounding streets with their cars and walked to the church, some parking nearly a mile away. Watching people file inside, I realized that nearly everyone I had ever known was here at this location, in honor of my mother. Mum always joked that she wanted her funeral to be "bombed out," that a full house at a funeral symbolized a full life. I smiled inwardly, thinking that this crowd would have exceeded even her wildest expectations.

A lover of religious hymns, Mum handpicked most of the songs that were to be sung in her memory. While I'd heard most of them countless times within those very walls with my mother, they took on entirely different meaning as I watched her casket wheeled down the center aisle. "Here I am Lord" opened the Mass. Distraught with grief, I lost all sense of my surroundings. The lyrics to this beautiful song were the only thing that registered. *"I who made the stars of night, I will make their darkness bright, Who will bear my light to them? Whom shall I send?"* The words went through me. The reference of light placed me back in the station wagon with Mum, waving at the rays of sunshine coming through the clouds. My mind was overwhelmed with emotion, and could only absorb fragmented thoughts and phrases. Make darkness bright…bear my light…angels…Mum. I was overcome. *"Here I am Lord. Is it I, Lord? I have heard you calling in the night. I will go, Lord, if you lead me. I will hold your people in my heart."* As the words rang out, I felt as if I was listening to them for the first time, and that they'd been written specifically for my mother. In a dreamlike state, I sat down as Father Al began my mother's service. The majority of the memorial, with the exception of the music, was a blur to me. Only during Holy Communion was my daze broken, as the church soloist serenaded the congregation with the song we'd chosen for Mum: "Wind Beneath My Wings." It was the single most hallowing rendition of the song I'd ever heard, and was the perfect dedication. *"It might have appeared to go unnoticed, but I've got it all here in my heart. I want you to know I know the truth…of course I know it…I would be nothing without you. Did you ever know that you're my hero? You're everything I wish I could be. I can fly higher than an eagle, 'cause you are the wind beneath my wings. Thank God for you, the wind beneath my wings."* Once again, the poignancy of the lyrics was indescribable, and unnervingly appropriate. I realized that as many times as I'd heard this song, I would never listen to it the same way again.

Suddenly I remembered that the conclusion of this ballad was my cue to approach the altar to read my eulogy. During the final refrain, I looked around me to see nearly everyone in tears. While he wasn't completely crying, even my little brother, who hadn't been able to express much emotion until that point, began to brim with heartache. Had I been required to read at any other point in the Mass, I most likely would not have been able. But the song had strengthened me. Bittersweet in its theme, "Wind Beneath My Wings" is an aria which commemorates how one person is empowered through the quiet strength of another. Mum had always held me up and allowed me to shine, and in doing so was deeply responsible for the person I had become and the person I would become. With this inspiration in my heart, I ascended the altar.

Placing my hand on Mum's casket as I exited the pew, I prayed for just a fraction of her courage to allow me to eulogize her properly. When I reached the pulpit, I turned and faced a magnificent sight. At first glance, I couldn't breathe, and thought I would be rendered speechless by awe. My shock quickly turned to vitalization, however, as I looked out on a church bursting at its seams with people who loved my mother. Not even on Christmas or Easter, when Masses were filled with "holiday Catholics," had I seen a bigger crowd in Immaculate. Packed from side to side, every seat on every bench was taken. The back hall was filled with people, and those who couldn't find a spot to sit or a place in the rear of the church lined themselves up the side aisles on both sides of the church, from front to back. I was overcome with pride, and had never felt so honored to do something in my life. My whole world was in that church, and had come to remember my mother. There was no greater venue in which to tell everyone I knew exactly how much I loved her, how much I would miss her, and how much she meant to me. More importantly, it was my opportunity before my friends, my family, and God, to honor my mother by sharing these sentiments with her.

While simple and grammatically incorrect, I have never written a more honest and heartfelt piece as this poem for my mother. For that reason, I have chosen not to alter it in any way. The following is the eulogy I wrote for her the day after she died.

I Wish You Could Have Been Here

I wish you could have been here, to see these people cry.
We cry because we love you so much, that's the reason why.
I wish you could have been here, to see Matthew drive his
first car.

But now you're where you deserve to be,
up in Heaven with Pa.

I wish you could have been here, to see Jimmy's graduation.
But I know you're glad you won't be here
for Clinton's Inauguration.

I wish you could have been here, to see me
walk down the aisle.

But I know when I think of you that day, you will surely
make me smile.

I wish you could have been here, to see Dad finally retire.

Because you will always be the two people I most admire.

I wish you could have been here, to see how beautiful
Grammy looks today.

I hope you realize how much happiness you brought
to all of us each day.

I wish you could have been here, so we could have
grown old together.

All the memories I have of you, I'll treasure them forever.

But now I realize something, most importantly,

That you really aren't gone, you're here...
standing right next to me.

And I realize something Mum, that you're here spiritually.

That you'll always be with the people who love you.

You'll always be with me.

I know we'll meet again one day, in a far better place.

And I can't wait to see that smile of yours, on that
beautiful, beautiful face.

But what made me most proud, until the very end,

Was the pleasure of having you for my very best friend.

Thank you Mum. We love you.

—Melin

While I kept my composure through most of the reading, my voice cracked with emotion as I read the final lines. I looked up at my dad and brothers to see them all crying, including Matthew. Walking back to them in silence, I kissed my hand and placed it on Mum's casket for the last time, and said goodbye to the physical.

CHAPTER 23

Praying Hands

THE FUNERAL PROCESSION TOOK US TO ST. JOSEPH'S CEMETERY IN WEST Roxbury, Massachusetts, where my mother was to be buried. Our limousine was filled with Mum's brothers and sisters, as well as my grandmother. I was thankful for their company on this somber ride. While I can't imagine what we were talking about, my aunts and uncles kept a light conversation going for the length of the journey. All discourse halted, however, when we arrived at the graveyard. We sat in silence in the parked limo for what seemed like an eternity. Squished between my father and my uncles, I could not see much of what was going on outside. Suddenly I heard my Aunt Sally from the back of the car. "Oh my God," she whispered under her breath. As I turned to follow her gaze, I saw the undertakers carrying my mother's casket from the hearse. Covered with overcoats and gloves, they struggled to climb over piles of snow to transport her body to the gravesite. As this harsh reality unfolded in front of my eyes, I once again began to cry. I couldn't believe what I was seeing. *I am about to bury my mother,* I thought, desperate with sadness. Sally, who had been sitting behind me, leaned forward and put her hands around me. "It's ok, Sweetheart," she said, as she herself came to tears. While practically nothing could have consoled me at that moment, her gentle touch gave me solace. As she very much had been in my mother's life, my aunt now also served as an angel in mine.

My dad, my brothers, and I were the first to reach the grave, followed closely by Mum's immediate family. Because the procession which tailed us from the church was nearly a mile long, we had an abundance of time to look upon the grievous sight in front of us. Though initially averting my eyes from the scene, I eventually forced myself to look at it in an effort of acceptance. Nonetheless, it was unbearable. At that point the casket had very much become a symbol of morbidity to me, and I needed to focus elsewhere. Suddenly my eyes were caught, for the first, time, by my mother's gravestone. While probably not the best object on which to fixate, especially as I was trying to escape the solemnity of death, Mum's headstone captivated me. It was unique in color, with a slight tint of rose which provided a sense of warmth compared to the various grey stones by which it was surrounded. Almost instantly, my view was drawn downward to the inscriptions on the grave:

Marian F. Ciampa 1948-1993

James. J. Ciampa, Jr. 1948-

Simultaneously, I felt the terminality of my mother's life span as well as the finiteness of my father's all in one glance. It was a sobering vision. I looked up at Dad, who was standing next to me, and cringed at the thought of having to return here one day to bury him with Mum. Staring at him, I went into denial. *He's right here. You're looking at him. You can touch him. He's not going anywhere*. But the actuality of what I had just gone through with my mother overpowered me. I began to privately panic. The idea of losing my father was brutally intolerable, and intensified by the circumstances. The events of the past few days and weeks were reaching their climax, and for a moment I thought I would not be able to make it through this final ceremony. As remaining mourners settled in around us and Father Al began reading passages from the Bible, I became blinded with tears. It was so final. Regardless of all the beautiful things my mother had passed on to me regarding the soul and the insignificance of physicality, I was debilitated by the conclusiveness of this event. Through watery eyes, I could see the hole beneath Mum's casket in which she would be placed. The thought of her being lowered into the ground sickened me. In the distance, I saw maintenance workers lingering around a bulldozer, patiently waiting for the crowd to disperse so they could bury my mother in that damned grave. I wanted to kill them. As a gradual rage built inside me, I began to cry even more intensely. Within moments, I felt someone gently slip a tissue into my hand. Thankful for this anonymous friend, I bowed my head and slowly wiped my face dry. As I lifted my eyes, I was taken off guard by an object on the gravestone which I had previously overlooked. There, in the center of the monument, was a set of praying hands. Beautifully crafted in copper, they were the focal point of the headstone. Always a favorite of Mum's, this symbol represented prayer and sincerity. Nothing could have been more appropriate, as my mother worshipped God in a fundamentally genuine manner. Her relationship with Him was based not in routine or rites; it was based in prayer. The simplicity of those hands, and what they symbolized, was very emblematic of my mother's life. As I looked at the image, I realized that the very object that had terrified me, the gravestone, contained an element in which I found peace. Had it not been for those hands, I'm sure I would have collapsed with grief. I focused on them for the remainder of the service. I believe they held me up that day, and I trust Mum made sure of it.

After the final blessing was read and our friends and family filed away, I stood with Dad and my brothers and said a final farewell to my mother. Seeing that I was struggling to leave, my father eventually put his arm around me and started to lead me back toward the car. "Come on, Pumpkin…it's ok," he said. I couldn't move. I couldn't say goodbye. Paralyzed, I closed my eyes and heard Mum's voice. *Keep me with you.*

Once again strengthened by her memory, I looked upon her casket for the final time and placed my hand over my heart. "I promise, Mum" I whispered, as I turned and walked away.

CHAPTER 24

The Gift

The Gift

By Melinda Marian Ciampa

Published in "The Cairn," Stonehill College literary magazine. Spring, 2000

Rays of Grace

My mum visited me the other night.
She sat right next to me,
Those rose-tinted cheeks still radiating life
from her beautiful face.
It was as if she'd never left.
I asked her what Heaven was like.
She told me that in order to explain what Heaven was like,
She had to first explain what life was like.
"Life is like a gift,
Boxed up in multiple layers.
You open one box only to find another,
And another, and another.
With each layer you open,
You reach a different level in your life,
One closer to fine, closer to the truth,
Closer to the gift.
With each layer you open,
You reach a new level of existence,
Realizing the interconnectedness of it all,
The purpose of life becomes clearer to you.
Some people have fewer boxes to open than others,
And reach their gifts before those around them.
These people understand the meaning of the gift
before most do,
And therefore receive it "early."
An accomplishment, not a punishment.
Those who take longer to open their gifts
Simply have more to unwrap before they receive.
But regardless of how long it takes,
And how many boxes have to be opened,
We all strive toward the same gift.
When you've reached every level you were meant to reach,
When you've realized everything you were meant to realize,
When you've opened every layer of your life,
Then, you receive your gift—
And that's what Heaven is like, Sweetheart."

CHAPTER 25

Fate

April 1, 2006. Massachusetts General Hospital. Yawkey Building. Ninth Floor. Sitting in the waiting room, I began to tremble. The gift shop I had just passed, which sold wigs and bandanas and bathing suits with prosthetic breast moldings, seemed ominously prophetic. As much as I dreaded this day, I had always known it would eventually come. Sensing my anxiety, my husband took my hands in his. "It'll be ok, Sweetie. You're going to be fine," he said. Looking into his soulful eyes, I started to cry.

Suddenly, a door opened and a voice called out, "Melinda?" Quickly wiping my tears, I stood up. It was Gayun Chan-Smutko, the genetic counselor whom I had seen four weeks earlier. Highly perceptive, she immediately picked up on my uneasiness. She walked toward me and with subtlety, put her hand on my shoulder. "I know this is difficult," she whispered, looking directly into my eyes. "So we'll walk through it together, ok?" Calmed by her gentleness, I nodded in agreement. "Come with me," Gayun then said, as she led me and my husband down the hallway.

Preparing myself to hear the results I somehow always knew I would receive, I inwardly began planning for the future. *You can handle this Melin. You always knew this day would come. Mum never had this opportunity. This way, you'll know ahead of time and be able to do something about it beforehand. You can plan your surgery for the fall; that way you can wear baggy clothes in the winter and your mastectomy might not be as obvious. Your life isn't over. You're only twenty-seven years old. This is just something you're going to have to deal with. It's just another chapter in your life.* I was about to receive the results of the hereditary cancer genetic testing I'd had performed a month earlier. Thirteen years had passed since Mum died, and thanks to amazing technological advancements, I was able to receive a test called BRACAnalysis, which was quickly becoming the standard of care in identifying individuals with hereditary breast and ovarian cancers. While thankful that this science had been developed, as I believed it would empower me with time and knowledge and options that were not afforded to my mother when she was diagnosed, I was also internally petrified. I was taken off guard by my nervousness. Since Mum had passed, I'd matured into a young woman with extreme passion and optimism toward life. My attitude was frighteningly similar to that of the woman from whom I'd inherited it. My faith was strong and my perspective in tact. Why, then, was I so scared? Perhaps it was the tumor I'd had removed from my breast eight years earlier. Although benign, I believed it to be an imminent foreshadowing of more serious things to come. Before I could reason with myself, my counselor interceded. "Unless you have any further questions, I'm going to cut right to the chase," she said, holding my test results in her hands. Once again, my husband Chris grabbed my hand in support. With a deep breath, I nodded my head. "I'm ready," I said. After opening and quickly gazing down at the piece of paper in her hands, Gayun looked at me and smiled. "Your results came back negative. 100% negative." Still holding the breath I had taken, and in partial shock, I had to double check that I'd heard her correctly. "Negative?" I asked. "Negative as in 'bad' or negative as in 'not present'?" Laughing lightheartedly, she explained. "Negative as in there were no mutations found in your DNA, which means that you're at no higher risk for breast cancer than anyone in general population. While this doesn't mean that you're completely off the hook… there are environmental links to the disease, so you will have to continue to screen yourself and get regular check ups as you have been…we found no hereditary genetic mutation related to breast cancer." As I tried to register her words, Chris sighed in relief. "I knew it, Babe," he said, kissing me on the forehead. Still I remained unresponsive, and unable to speak. Gayun retranslated the information, as she could see my disbelief. "This is good news, Melinda," she said. "Again, it doesn't mean you're not at risk at all, but your risk is a heck of a lot lower than it would have been had we found a genetic connection." Exhaling finally, I felt purified. What I had come to accept as my fate was in fact not so. Not overlooking the fact that I would need to sustain my current methods of prevention, I just couldn't believe what I had heard. "I'm going to give you two a moment alone," Gayun said, reaching for the doorknob. "Oh…no, we're fine. There's no need to…." I started to say, in an effort to minimize the emotional significance of the moment. "It's ok," she continued. "Sometimes this sort of news is best absorbed in privacy." Placing the test results on the table, so I could read them with my own eyes, this wonderful lady then slipped quietly out of the room and gently shut the door behind her. Before it was fully closed, I burst into tears of happiness in my husband's arms. *Thank you, Mum,* I thought, as my soul breathed easily.

CHAPTER 26

Survival

THE DEFINITION OF A SURVIVOR IS A PERSON WHO CONTINUES TO FUNCTION or prosper in spite of opposition, hardship, or setbacks. While my mother ultimately died of breast cancer, she fulfills this description possibly better than any other person I've known. Though her body may have eventually given out, her perseverance did not. Throughout her life, Mum's spirit stood in defiance of adversity and affliction. It is on account of her example, in life and in dying, that my family has survived. Through our duration as a family, her soul and legacy continue to flourish. Hence, my mother survives.

Having lost Mum when I was fourteen, I could fill another book with stories from having grown up without her. My father, my brothers and I ate Hungry Man dinners for about two years until Dad thankfully learned how to cook a couple meals. Then we ate those for two years, but were more than grateful to not have frozen food every night. Because he sympathized with us, my father grew more lenient in certain aspects. While he still disciplined us, he didn't obsess over things like curfews or strict codes of conduct. He focused simply on raising us, as best he could, to be good kids. That's it... just kind and decent kids. There are endless accounts that could be shared from this transitional period; some sad, some hilarious, and some unbelievable. And while we may have suffered a few more scratches than the average family along the way, we all evolved into people of whom I think my mother would be very proud.

Dad remarried about four years after Mum passed. Brief in its duration, the marriage lasted only a year, at which point both he and his wife realized it wasn't meant to be. Shortly after his divorce, my father underwent open-heart surgery to replace his aortic valve. While my mother's influence taught me not to fear my own death, the experience of having lost her made me undeniably terrified of losing Dad. Thankfully he not only survived the procedure, he gained a newfound perspective on his own life. In doing so, my father redefined his priorities and found happiness. In 2004 he remarried again, this time getting it right. His wife, Lee, aside from being one of the nicest people I've ever met, is wonderful for my father. Although he has been known to drive her up a wall on occasion, Dad loves her deeply and has very much found a true companion. The addition of Lee and her daughters, Stephanie and Kim, to our family has truly been a gift, and has enhanced my life greatly.

Jimmy entered the military after high school, and eventually went on to earn a degree in business, putting himself through college while working full time. A far cry from the shy little boy who used to get picked on in school, my older brother has become quite a man. Now frighteningly strong, he has the build my father had at his age. With a combination of good looks and sociability, Jim never had any trouble attracting women. Though he dated incessantly throughout his teens and early twenties, he ended up marrying his first love Allison, whom he met when he was eighteen. He's one of the people I respect most in the world.

Matt graduated in the top of his class in both high school and college, and is now leading a successful life in Miami, Florida. As Mum predicted, he became my confidant and dearest friend. The best listener I've ever known, "Rat" (as I call him) has been my personal therapist since we were kids. Just like his mother, he has a keen sense of when just to listen and when to give advice. No matter what, he has never judged me, and for this I am immeasurably grateful. His counsel and friendship have been staples in my life, and I attribute much of my personal development to him. Our relationship is one of my most sacred possessions.

And how has my life turned out, you ask? Sincerely blessed. I've achieved a level of happiness greater than I ever thought attainable, thanks largely in part to an angel who walked into my world *"when I least expected it."* While no words can aptly express how deeply he has beautified my existence, my husband Chris is, quite simply, the love of my life. Possessing quiet strength and extraordinary gentleness, he is the best man I've ever known, and my best friend. His love will fill the pages of my life. Besides having found this radiant soul, I have very much enjoyed discovering myself as well. While I realize there is much more yet to be uncovered, I am truly happy with the woman whom I've unveiled so far. I have grown into a strong, passionate, intelligent woman. I have earned the respect of honest, honorable people. I have succeeded academically, personally, and professionally. And above all, I have a firm grasp of what is genuinely important to me: my family, my friends, my dignity, and my spirituality. While I am not without fault, I have done my best to be a loving person and treat others with kindness and compassion. Ultimately, the meaning in my life is found in these simplicities.

Today my family remains very close. Although we each now have our own lives and responsibilities, my father, my brothers, and I maintain our core relationship. We have come to a point in our lives at which we can truly enjoy one another. The distance which separates us simultaneously compels us to appreciate the time we have together. Ironically, it is my family's "imperfections," the things which either bothered me as a child or that which I felt needed improvement, which have become most treasured to me. Although we have all considered ourselves to be dysfunctional at some point, I think we've realized that we did the best we could have with the hand we were dealt. While our lives have not been perfect, so neither have anyone else's been. We've come to learn that no one has a "normal" family; that everyone, to varying degrees, bears his own cross. And though we've endured the tragedy of my mother's death, we have survived, and are stronger as a result of it. This is who we are; we are a family, and through everything, we have taken care of each other. As Mum would have wished.

Chapter 27

Snapshots

About a year ago, I had a conversation with my brother Matthew which further enhanced my understanding of life. One of many such dialogues we've had throughout the years, this particular talk centered on the significance of memories, and the specific moments that serve to change and define our time here. "If you think about it, Melin, all we'll have at the end of our lives is a series of snapshots; mental pictures we've taken which will remind us of where we've been and what we've experienced in this world," he said. "Although some images may be more vivid and prominent than others, your collection will be uniquely your own, and will ultimately be your testament to life." As I conceptualized his theory, I tried to imagine what transparencies I would most readily recall on my deathbed. While some of the greatest moments in life occur in momentous occasions, others are cultivated in complete privacy. In my own existence, the latter have proven to be the most beautiful.

One such example was in fact a very paramount moment: the day my husband proposed to me. The date was March 29, 2003. Chris and I had been dating for four years. Although spring had officially arrived, winter had been extending its stay, as often the case in New England. The forecast for this day, however, was encouraging. Expecting the first decent weather of the season, my boyfriend and I headed north to the seacoast of New Hampshire to take a walk along the beach and grab lunch in Portsmouth. To our initial dismay, the conditions were not as predicted. It was overcast and about forty degrees outside. But thanks to an innate understanding of dressing in layers, and driven by a hunger to get to the coast, we proceeded with our planned trip. We parked along an empty side road across from the beach. As we strolled toward the ocean, I expressed my joy in the situation. "I love t-shirt and jeans days," I said, commenting on our casualness. Grinning knowingly, Chris agreed. As we reached the shore, I bounced toward the surf and began to step dance on the sand, while my sweetheart skipped rocks into the water. Due to the temperature and the time of year, Chris and I had the beach to ourselves. It was our playground. Rejoicing in the elements, I looked upward as I inhaled a deep breath of salt water air. My eyes were met unexpectedly by one of my favorite visions in life; rays of sunshine delicately coming through the clouds. Breathless, I turned to see if Chris had noticed this gorgeous display. He was one of the few people with whom I'd shared the significance of this representation, and how I'd come to learn of it through Mum. As I looked at him, his gaze came downward from the sky and fixated on me. No words were needed. Without speaking, he simply smiled, intuitively aware of my emotions. Wanting to get the perfect view, I climbed onto a giant rock which was partially submerged in the low tide. Chris followed moments after. With each passing wave, it seemed more and more beams of light poured from the heavens. Wrapping his arms around me from behind, my love whispered into my ear. "Your mum is with us right now," he said, squeezing me gently. "I know," I replied, as I welled with sentiment. As I stared in awe at the horizon, I felt true happiness. I had found my angel, the man who respected me, loved me, and understood me on a level few others ever would. How appropriate that my ultimate angel was here, shining down on me in my elation. "I want to be here with you when we're old and grey," Chris said as he kissed the side of my face. "Me too, Babe," I answered, as I turned to meet his lips. Before I was fully rotated, Chris took my hand and bent down on his right knee. As he held up my wedding ring for me to see for the very first time, his eyes filled with tears. "Will you marry me, Sweetie?" With the warmth of grace on my back, and overwhelmed with joy, I broke down crying as I accepted. We celebrated quietly and passionately in each others arms for several minutes before turning back toward the sea. Feeling the radiance of the sun, we realized that we were no longer only looking at the sunbeams in the distance, but we were now standing directly inside of one's path. "Best seat in the house," we said simultaneously. As we beheld one another in endearment of our synchronization, I could not quantify the happiness I felt in knowing I would spend the rest of my life with this beautiful soul. Though our wedding day occurred several months later, our marriage was blessed that very day on the beach. As promised, Mum hadn't missed a single moment.

Another cherished memory, which took place in complete privacy and years after she had passed, enlightened me further to my mother's character. Almost two years had gone by since Mum's death, and Dad had finally brought himself to clean out her belongings. Her closet was still filled with her clothing, and her vanity still housed her fragrances and medication. My father had asked me to go through my mother's belongings and take whatever

I wanted before he offered anything to my aunts and family. I had already taken her perfume shortly after she died. Not to ever wear it myself, but so I could keep her with me in some earthly sense. It eventually evaporated, I believe from my smelling it so often. After gathering some clothes and jewelry, I looked inside the "junk" drawer in her bureau to see if I could find any trinkets. In it, I found everything from old Mother's Day cards my brothers and I had written her, to gimp bracelets we'd made in camp, to a scribbled piece of paper with a song I'd composed on it. It seemed as if she'd kept everything we'd ever given her. As I searched further, I found several stacks of pictures which captured different phases of Mum's life. There was a photograph of her and my father making out in a parking lot the night they met (I knew this because I recognized the dress she was wearing in the picture. She had kept it and rarely wore it again after that night). She'd held on to pictures of Jimmy, Matt, and me playing on the beach down the Cape. The seagulls in the backgrounds of these shots made me shake my head with silent laughter. Then I came across photos I'd never seen before. They were close-up self-portraits of my mother, which she must have taken by holding the camera in front of her own face. The first image was of Mum in her soft red turban, which she wore when she lost her hair during chemotherapy. She was looking directly into the lens and was uncharacteristically straight-faced. The second print stopped me in my tracks, as it revealed something on which I had never laid my eyes: Mum's bald head. Again, she had never allowed my brothers or me to see her without hair in an effort to reduce the impact of her cancer treatment on us. I believe she did this as an act of protection, and to keep our lives as normal as possible. As I stared at the picture, I wondered what her intention was in taking such a photo. Once again, her countenance was serious. Flipping one further into the stack, I viewed practically the same picture, only this time Mum was grinning ear to ear. I smiled inwardly as I gazed upon my friend in her most natural expression. Finally,

I turned to the last photo in the pile. Sporting her most classic goofy Marian face, complete with crossed eyes, twisted jaw, and tongue hanging out, my mother had snapped one final shot of herself. The consummate joker, Mum was very animated, and famous for making silly faces like this. My heart swelled with enjoyment upon this sight. *She meant for this to happen exactly as it just did,* I thought to myself. Mum knew I would eventually find those photographs, and I believe she took them and strategically placed them where I would discover them. I could almost hear her talking to me. *Here I am, Sweetie. I'm still here. Still laughing and still smiling. It's safe for you to see me this way now. I'm not sick anymore. I'm ok.* Standing alone in her room, holding her memory in my hands and moreover in my heart, I experienced one of the most intimate moments I ever shared with my mother.

Each in its own way, these occasions marked my life. They allowed me to experience Heaven within everyday occurrences, and empowered me to continue my relationship with Mum. Snapshots such as these, the most private and sacred in my collection, will be with me when I prepare for my own divine transition. As I realize these images constitute just glimpses of what has made my life so beautiful, I hope to fill my scrapbook with similar memories which I've yet to encounter or imagine. After all, if it's the only possession I'm allowed to take with me to the next life, I better make it good.

CHAPTER 28

Rays of Grace

MY MOTHER USED TO SAY THAT PEOPLE WHO GO THROUGH LIFE without experiencing any sort of hardship have more difficulty recognizing goodness because they are desensitized to it. They lack counterbalance. On the contrary, individuals who have endured tragedy can typically identify moments of joy more readily, even in the most subtle of circumstances. It's a matter of attitude. American writer Charles Swindoll once said, "Life is ten percent what happens to you and ninety percent how you react to it." I could have easily imploded in self-pity after my mother's death, but instead I accepted the situation and adapted to it. I'd be lying if I said it wasn't difficult. Without a doubt, it was the greatest pain I've ever suffered. There is a difference, however, between feeling sad and feeling sad for oneself. Had I not taken

Rays of Grace

all the time I needed to properly mourn and recognize my loss, my healing process would have been drastically different, as I would be. I've found that channeling my journey through grief toward finding peace, rather than attaining closure, has been a vital part of my evolution. Perhaps most critical, however, is the inspiration I found in my mum. In all the adversity she faced, she never once complained. No matter how grim the situation, she never failed to find the silver lining within it.

Take for instance, my mother's diagnosis of breast cancer. Within the multiple conversations we had in the hospital during the last weeks of her life, my mother shared a perspective I never would have imagined had it not been for her unique outlook. "There's nothing in the world I wouldn't trade to have my health back, Sweetie, but it's just not in the cards," she said. "It took me a while, but I've come to terms with it. So what am I going to do now...bitch about it? What good is that going to do? I'd rather spend my time thinking about the good things that have transpired as a result of this whole ordeal." Although I understood her stance on not complaining, I could not imagine to what good she was possibly referring. "Like what?" I asked innocently. As Mum smiled, I could see her drift into different scenarios in her mind. "Had I never become ill, I would have never gotten my drinking under control, and your father and I would most likely be separated. We're closer now than we've ever been." With one simple sentence, my mother enlightened me to a different way of perception. I had never even stopped to think about these possibilities. I had only focused on the negative. As I absorbed the impact of her words, she continued. "And while I'd give anything to have more time with you Melin, at least we've had the opportunity to say goodbye to one another and have these conversations. Some people never have that chance. Dad lost his father suddenly to a heart attack. He never had this luxury. If you think of it that way, this is a blessing which few others ever receive. " Once again, Mum provided me with a new set of eyes

127

with which to view the world. While I had been hard pressed to find anything optimistic about her terminal condition, she succeeded in giving me something in which to believe.

Finally, Mum commented on the importance of appreciating the balance of life. "God works in mysterious ways, Sweetie. There will be times when you'll experience so much happiness you won't even know what to do with yourself. It will seem as if you have the world in the palm of your hand. There will also be things that happen in your life which you won't understand; things that won't seem fair; things that won't work out the way you intend. Although you may not realize it until years later, they will have happened for a reason. There are no mistakes and no accidents. It's often the case that the thing you don't plan on, the thing you least expect, might be the best thing that ever happens to you. It might be a ray of grace. That's why you have to embrace life in its entirety; the good and the bad. You can't take one without the other, as they are both equally significant. Each will offer you something meaningful from which you'll have the opportunity to learn and develop as a human being. It's what you decide to do with the time and circumstances you're given that will define your life. That choice will always be yours, Sweetie. That's why I'll never worry about you. You've always been able to see the sunshine through the clouds."

Reminiscing fourteen years later on my mother's words, I can't help but envision that gorgeous fall afternoon, when she first introduced me to a new understanding of angels. Since that day, every single time I've seen rays of sunshine coming through the clouds, I've waved at them. As you'd imagine, this spectacle has become even more sacred to me since Mum died, as I now see her in those sunbeams. In addition to providing me with heightened sentimental significance, this phenomenon has also awakened me to the power of contrast. Having admired these displays closely, I have come to appreciate the integral role darkness plays in enhancing the beauty of light. The vision of beams of sunshine pouring down through the heavens is one of the most spectacular in nature, but its beauty would be diminished without the contraposition between the clouds and sunlight. Each intensifies the other's effect, and in doing so accentuates the overall exquisiteness of the sight. Hence, the very essence of this display lies within balance and distinction. The clouds are equally as important as the sun; darkness as critical as light. Just as my mother had explained the week before she passed, each has a harmonious purpose. Similarly, I've come to acknowledge and understand the significance of hardship and darkness in my own life. As a result, everything else in my world has become that much more beautiful.

One last thought on sunshine. By its nature, it's invisible. While we have clear sight of the things which it illuminates, we can't actually see sunshine itself. But we know it's there. We can feel it on our faces on a summer day. Likewise, we can often see the effect it has on people. Sometimes its presence alone is enough to make someone's day more enjoyable. Amazing for something that isn't tangible, isn't it? In fact the only time we can see sunshine is when it's accentuated by darkness, as when it shines through the clouds. It seems that angels and sunshine go hand in hand. While they're not always perceivable, they still very much exist. I've learned to look with my eyes and see with my heart, and in doing so have realized that the most important things in life are invisible. I never asked Mum how she knew about the angels that waved down to us from the sky that day. Looking back, I think I've figured it out. Perhaps it takes an angel, to know one.

"Unexpected moments of grace are often bestowed upon us by angels attempting to awaken our souls."

Acknowledgments

THE AUTHOR WOULD LIKE TO THANK ROBERT J. MCEWAN, EDITOR AND friend, under whose mentorship I realized my love of writing; Kevin Penwell, for opening the door; my father Jim and my brothers Jimmy and Matt, for being the men they are and for always protecting me. Thank you for allowing me to write a truly authentic piece. My deep appreciation to my husband Chris, who listened to these stories well before they were ever written. For laughing and crying with me throughout this beautiful journey, and for your undying encouragement and support, thank you Sweetheart. Finally, my ultimate gratefulness to my mum, Marian Ciampa, whose love and laughter have made my life.

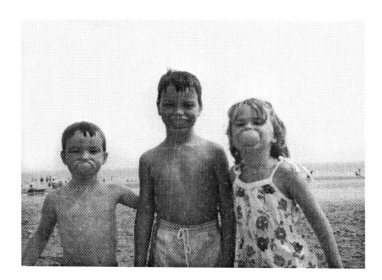

Onset Beach - 1984

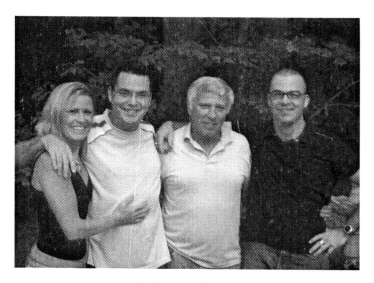

Melinda, Matt, Dad, Jimmy

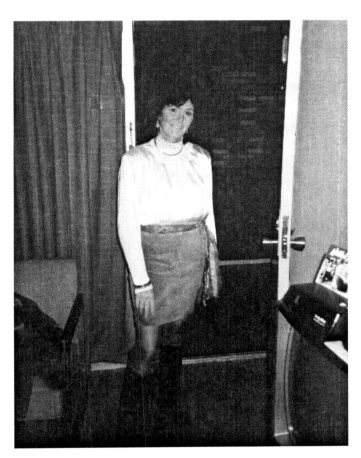

Mum. Eternally beautiful

About the Author

Born and raised in Boston, Massachusetts, Melinda Marian Ferreira developed an early love of literature and poetry when she discovered the works of New Englanders such as Ralph Waldo Emerson, Henry David Thoreau, and Robert Frost. Profoundly inspired by the sense of connection she felt within their words, she was compelled to write from a very early age. A firm believer that the power of such expression transcends

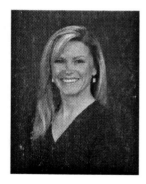

Author Melinda Ferreira

time and place, Melinda's influences are based in writings that cultivate human connection and understanding, whether through stories, poetry, or song. In an effort to promote awareness, healthy development and well being, Melinda works closely with centers for grieving children, breast cancer organizations, and alcoholism programs on both regional and national levels. She lives with her husband, Chris, on the Seacoast of New Hampshire.